n=1

How the Uniqueness of
Each Individual Is
Transforming Healthcare

How the Uniqueness of Each Individual Is
Transforming Healthcare

John Koster, M.D.
Former CEO, Providence Health & Services

Gary Bisbee, Ph.D.
Chairman and CEO, The Health Management Academy

Ram Charan
Co-author of *Execution: The Discipline of Getting Things Done*

The Academy Press

AND

PROSPECTA PRESS

Published by
The Academy Press
in association with Prospecta Press
An imprint of Easton Studio Press
P.O. Box 3131
Westport, CT 06880
(203) 571-0781
www.prospectapress.com

Book design by Barbara Aronica-Buck

Hardcover ISBN: 978-1-63226-018-5
E-book ISBN: 978-1-63226-019-2

Printed in the United States of America
Second printing March 2015

CONTENTS

PART I

The Culture
of Questions

Knowledge is having the right answer.
Wisdom is having the right question.
—Author unknown

Our experience with leaders of successful organizational transformation underscores the importance of incisive questions and inquiry. This begins with the leader's self-reflection and personal inquiry. What does change mean to me? How must I change? How do I feel about that? Deep understanding of the environment is then gained through fearless inquiry in and out of the organization, especially with customers. The successful leaders cultivate an organizational culture of inquisitiveness. In uncertain times, incisive questioning is the best way for organizations to learn. Answering questions is learning. Answering the best questions leads to the best choices.

CHAPTER 1

Healthcare Transformation and the Importance of Questions

Shortly before the passage of the Patient Protection and Affordable Care Act (ACA), there was a dialogue among a group of healthcare CEOs. They were asked if there would be a transformation of healthcare even if the ACA didn't pass. The leaders uniformly responded that the ACA could be a factor; however, other forces were causing healthcare to be transformed, regardless of the passage of the ACA. At that time, they saw the impact of the ACA as uncertain, but the forces of transformation were undeniable. Since its passage, the ACA has variably influenced all sectors of healthcare. However, as those healthcare leaders correctly predicted, the transformation of healthcare has accelerated, well beyond the impact of the ACA.

Healthcare Transformation

The underlying catalysts for healthcare transformation are digitization and scientific innovation, both of which, by their nature, are disruptive. The impact of these forces on healthcare is amplified by the societal reality of unsustainable healthcare costs at historical growth rates. These healthcare costs are driving the transference of risk. This risk transference is seen in health benefit and payment model changes.

The most dramatic influence of the transformational forces is on individuals. Access to information accelerates the desire of individuals to act, behave, and be treated uniquely. Individuals have choices and options in every aspect of their lives. Access to more and timely information increases their options. Individuals will choose the option most suited to their unique needs. This is what we mean by "n = 1" and why we titled the book accordingly.

The n = 1 symbolizes our uniqueness as individuals in today's digitized world. The expression n = 1 is used in mathematics and computer programming to ask the question "How many?" In this book, "n" represents persons; thus, the notation n = 1 refers to an individual. The n = 1 represents a biologically, psychologically, and sociologically unique individual. Throughout the world, each person, using his resources and capabilities, chooses options that fit his unique needs, which we refer to as n = 1.

The impact of the n = 1, powered by the disruption caused by digitization and scientific innovation, cannot be overstated. It is changing every aspect of our global lives through interconnectivity, social networking, democratization of information, and increasing customization of products and services. Most industries have already undergone levels of transformation, and some have been profoundly changed or rendered obsolete.

Healthcare transformation is in its infancy, but it is unstoppable. It is beginning to influence and will soon create havoc in the structure and in the competitive landscape of the healthcare industry. Let us be clear, given the current pace of transformation, that the skills needed to lead healthcare organizations will be dramatically different in the future.

The term "transformation" can be overused, but it is not in this instance. It describes healthcare's future without exaggeration. Transformation refers to the *fundamental* changes a business, profession, or industry must make in order to be successful when there is a shift in the market environment. Sometimes the shifts are easily seen, and the changes required are readily apparent. Other times the shifts are so profound and fundamental that their connection to the business environment can be difficult for leaders to see.

The n = 1, empowered by the transformative forces of digitization and scientific innovation, challenges the fundamental structure and assumptions of healthcare. The societal context of unsustainable healthcare costs and resulting changes in payment models further accelerate transformation. Healthcare leaders are looking deeply into the changes that are occurring, and they are identifying the fundamental structures and assumptions that are likely to be transformed.

Lessons from Other Industries

The n = 1 has already transformed many industries, if not most. A useful example is the music industry. The early peer-to-peer music file-sharing service Napster transformed the music industry more than a decade ago.[1] Through Napster, individuals could get the music they wanted, through their computer, and for free. Even in the early days of the Internet, this level of access to intellectual property seemed too good to be true. The flood of downloading MP3 files strained college computer networks. The music industry and recording artists took legal action against Napster; Napster lost many legal challenges and changed their systems, but the downloading continued. The music industry began legal action against individuals in an attempt to regain control of their product.

Individuals saw the opportunity to customize music for their unique desires. The coincident development of MP3 players allowed people to create their own playlists. When the music industry responded by suing its customers, leaders did not have a plan beyond defending their product. Music industry leaders could not imagine how they would maintain control in a world where consumers had such individualized choice and access to copyrighted music. Previously, production executives sitting in "smoke-filled rooms" selected fourteen songs for an album, forcing consumers to buy the entire lot even if they only wanted one or two songs. Following the introduction of Napster, album sales began a long, steady decline.

The whole process of the industry, from finding artists all the way through the distribution of the content via CD, was being challenged. The music industry did not "face the music." There were those entrepreneurs outside the industry who saw opportunity. They were unencumbered by the business model and by history. Apple filled the device niche with a stylish and easy-to-use MP3 player, the iconic iPod. Apple was not the first to enter the MP3 player market, but it provided a legal, easy-to-use music downloading service, iTunes. The game changed. The two transformative and disruptive components of the sale of music—digitization (commercialized as iTunes) and scientific innovation (sold as the iPod)—changed everything. The music industry didn't like it, but it had few alternatives.

Tastes and needs of the individual in music have continued to evolve. Pandora, Rhapsody, iTunes Radio, and Beats are but few of the digitally enabled alternatives for individuals to access music. We believe that the only organizations that continue to evolve with the demands and tastes of n = 1 will thrive.

The leaders of the music industry viewed the challenges of Napster as a legal issue. The changes were so fundamental that many leaders missed the tectonic shifts that were occurring. The questions regarding the fundamental and profound changes to the music industry were asked only in the context of their historic business model. Their customers, the n = 1, had changed.

What were the questions they should have asked? Legal issues certainly needed attention, but how could they have expanded their awareness of what was actually happening to the distribution of *all* intellectual property? Could they have responded by selling their own digital music? Could the industry have come together with collaborative, innovative organizations to bring the scale required to create their own digital marketplace?

"Music Industry to Abandon Mass Suits"
WSJ.com by Sarah McBride and Ethan Smith
Updated December 19, 2008, 12:01 a.m. ET

After years of suing thousands of people for allegedly stealing music via the Internet, the recording industry is set to drop its legal assault as it searches for more effective ways to combat online music piracy.

The decision represents an abrupt shift of strategy for the industry, which has opened legal proceedings against about 35,000 people since 2003. Critics say the legal offensive ultimately did little to stem the tide of illegally downloaded music. And it created a public relations disaster for the industry, whose lawsuits targeted, among others, several single mothers, a dead person, and a thirteen-year-old girl.

The Importance of Questions

The leadership challenge is to sense when and how the existing business model of a given industry must transform. People and organizations resist change. Successful leaders prepare their people and organizations in anticipation of change. The window of opportunity to successfully introduce change can be small. Leaders introduce change before not-changing becomes a dire situation. People act on the basis of avoiding pain, so producing change before the pain is felt is a leadership challenge.

The transformative and disruptive forces of digitization and scientific innovation are accelerating, but their effect on any given healthcare institution or community is unpredictable, particularly in the short term. Our research and experience confirm that, in situations of great uncertainty, the best leaders ask lots of questions.

Every healthcare organization is at a different point in its relationship to transformation. No two organizations have the same strategy, mission, and structure or the same market dynamic. One size does not fit all for healthcare organizations or markets. The uniqueness and diversity of healthcare organizations requires an individualized approach to transformation.

In our conversations with leaders in healthcare, there is a sense of things being turned topsy-turvy. These unsettled feelings extend to all levels of healthcare. The immediate challenge to just keep things on track is overwhelming, aside from thinking about transformation. This is not surprising. Even experienced executives report that the level of change is higher than at any other time in their careers. Uncertainty is the rule.

Successful leaders have a conceptual framework for the questions that will guide their organizations. This framework is drawn from training, experience, and formal education. We think of a framework as a tool or an approach that brings order and connection in an incredibly complex, fast-moving, and uncertain world. The conceptual framework should be high-level and easily understood.

A conceptual framework will provide a structure for dialogue and develop a commonality of understanding among the leadership, the organization, and the board of directors. The conceptual framework is a guide for interpreting events and asking questions about the future. It does not attempt to explain everything.

A conceptual framework for transformation has two parts. The first part is designed to understand the nature of the forces driving transformation. The second part focuses on understanding competencies and structures.

A conceptual framework "connects the dots" between the forces of transformation and organizational requirements. This book encompasses both the forces of transformation and the organizational requirements. It is a guide showing leaders how to begin to connect the dots. First, leaders socialize the conceptual framework; then they pursue incisive questioning.

Questions remain a most important tool for a leader engaged in transformative change. Questions are the driver for change, and the best leaders use rigor, intellectual honesty, and insight in shaping questions and interpreting answers. Answers to an identical question will vary from organization to organization and from leader to leader.

The human brain has a remarkable capacity to both ask and answer questions. This interaction of "Q and A" is what we call thinking. The brain will answer any question you choose to ask. If you ask poor questions such as "Why does this always happen to me?" your brain will work relentlessly to come up with reasons why this always happens to you. If you ask questions such as "What are the ways I can make this situation better?" your brain will work hard to answer that question. Just like each of us individually, organizations must ask the best questions possible. Leaders set the example for the questioning.

> "If I had an hour to solve a problem and my life depended on a solution, I would spend the first fifty-five minutes determining the proper question to ask, for, once I knew the proper question, I could solve the problem in less than five minutes."
>
> — Attributed to Albert Einstein

There are challenges for leaders asking questions. Change is stressful for organizations and leaders. There are some individuals who believe that the leader should always know everything. Leaders who ask a lot of questions may be perceived as weak or indecisive and may make people anxious. Outstanding leaders cultivate the art of asking incisive questions throughout their organization. They develop a culture of inquiry in their organizations, and clearly communicate the rationale that questions are the best approach to uncertainty.

Leaders coach, learn, and get to the core of complex situations through asking incisive questions, taking high-level concepts from 50,000 feet and, through a series of questions, developing understanding. It is an art, and, like any art, it is developed by practice.

So what do incisive questions look like, and what are they intended to accomplish?

Example of Incisive Questions

Tony, a health system CEO, is reviewing a plan by a local business to challenge and overtake the current leader in its market. The leader of the local business unit, Alan, is presenting the plan, along with four of his colleagues. Tony knows and respects the local team and views them as strong leaders in the health system. Tony wants them to be successful, but perhaps most of all he wants them to continue to develop their questioning, thinking, and judgment skills.

The meeting starts informally with Tony engaging them in informal conversation and relaxing the environment for the discussion. As the review begins, Tony says he does not want to see their PowerPoint presentation (they had over 100 slides prepared); he prefers to have a dialogue. Alan is pleased, as he always learns a lot from Tony's questions. Alan's team, on the other hand, is disappointed, that they won't be showing the boss their animated PowerPoint demonstration of how they will crush the competition.

The dialogue begins:

Tony: "What is the goal you want to accomplish in next four years?"

Alan: "Within that timeframe, we will move from number three to number one in market share, as well as in profitability.

Most leaders would follow up with the one-word question, "How?" Instead, Tony asks:

Tony: "From whom will you gain the market share?"

Alan: "From number one, the market leader."

Tony: "Let me be clear: what specific elements of number one's business will you take?"

Alan: "The large customer segment in which the number-one guy has 60 percent of the market share."

Most people would ask how you would gain that share. Instead, Tony asks:

Tony: "Tell us about customer behavior in that segment. What drives their purchasing decisions?"

Alan: "We will give them superior technology compared to the market leader."

Tony notes to himself that this answer did not respond to his question.

Tony: "When will the technology be ready?"

Alan: "Twenty-four months."

Tony: "What is your view of the technology competency of number one? How different will your technology offering have to be for the customer to pay? Will they pay not only for the technology, but also for the switching cost? By the way, you still haven't told me about the customer behavior and who the decision-maker is for those customer segments."

Alan: "I have the market research report; I can show you in that slide."

Tony: "Don't show me the slide. Tell me your professional judgment about the information on the slide. Lastly, how many customers did you personally interview?"

Tony's tone was that of a coach. He told the group that he would support their strategy, and advised them to do some more homework and come back in a few weeks. He specifically directed them to talk to the customers.

This vignette demonstrates the art of asking incisive questions. Like many skills, it is best cultivated through practice. It avoids generic questions. In this whole thirty-minute discourse, questions like how to gain competitive advantage were not asked. Penetrating questions that generated specific insights were posed. This is the skill that leaders should practice.

In times of transformation, the leader asks questions not merely to gather information. Because questions stimulate thinking, they are as much about generating different ways for the organization to view itself. Simple questions designed simply to gather information are important, but they may not move the organization forward in its thinking. Incisive questions are designed to stimulate dialogue and reveal underlying assumptions that can either help or hinder transformation.

The Nokia Example

The Nokia board's interaction with a new CEO several years ago[2] is illustrative of questions that accomplish more than simply gathering facts.

Early in the days of wireless handsets, Nokia was a market leader. The management suspected that Apple would be entering the market. Apple had over 200 patents that would be directly relevant to innovative new wireless platforms. For a host of reasons, Nokia did not respond successfully. They had seen the Apple iPhone coming; they had all the clues, but they did not respond. The board ultimately replaced the CEO when they saw they were unprepared for the transformation of the industry.

The new CEO came from Microsoft and had experience in software development. The board of directors asked the incoming CEO to review the organization and assess the situation, with a plan to get together and review in ninety days.

What would be the questions the board should ask after the assessment?

They would include: How is cash flow? What is your assessment of the management team? What are your goals and priorities? Then the board would move to understand the assumptions that underpinned the approach to making the company competitive in the new landscape. How would it transform? Their current product is not technologically competitive in the more sophisticated markets.

The board asked: What is your current view of the compelling customer needs, and how will customer need be different by the time you're ready to launch your new product? How will the iPhone change customers' expectations by the time you launch your product? Define the specifications of the consumer experience for your new product. What will be the customer experience for the iPhone model you expect to be in place when you launch?

Further, what are the specifics about the launch of the new product that will reposition it positively against the iPhone? What are the specific reasons you think you will build a product with features that

> "Stephen Elop's Nokia Adventure"
> by Peter Burrows, *Bloomberg Business Week*, June 2, 2011
>
> Nokia's initial reaction to the iPhone is the most embarrassing example of what went wrong. When Steve Jobs unveiled the device in January 2007, "it was widely disregarded," says former manager Dave Grannan, who now runs [the] Burlington (Mass.)-based voice recognition company Vlingo. "The attitude was that we'd tried touch-screens before, and people didn't like them." It had no multimedia messaging (MMS) capability. The reception and sound quality were poor. It couldn't be used with one hand. There was nothing to fear.
> As iPhone sales took off, Nokia remained strangely detached, say a dozen current and former executives. The company didn't sit still, exactly. It opened its own app store, Ovi—but never put marketing muscle behind it. With no runaway hit like the iPhone, app developers largely ignored it. When CEO Elop euthanized the Ovi brand name on May 16, it had 50,000 apps; Apple had 500,000. "It was an ignorant complacency, not an arrogant complacency," says Nokia human resources head Juha Akras.

will generate market movement from the iPhone? What about other competitors, like Samsung? Do you have the right talent to execute this strategy with urgency and dedication? Is your talent as good as or better than Apple's? To support the new product, do you have relationships with others not in the company, like the app developer community, that you will need? What are your milestones? What specifically should we look at to assess your progress?

This line of questioning is not the only way to get to the point. It's up to each leader to develop a style of inquiry. These exercises highlight the fact that this is not a battle of PowerPoint presentations. This is a dialogue of give-and-take, with exploration of assumptions to develop insight and common understanding.

It is often helpful to use a few simple sketches or diagrams to illustrate key points, and, in the sessions of inquiry, to recall that different people listen, see, and learn in very different ways.

Board members, after this dialogue, were able to more fully understand the new CEO's plan and to gain insight into their organization's assumptions about transformation. The plan was based on the CEO's conceptual framework of market transformation driven by the iPhone. Their questions deepened their understanding of how the CEO was connecting the opportunities for transformation with the changes required in Nokia competencies and organization.

The story of the CEO and board after this interchange is beyond the scope of this book, but it is a useful study about an attempted turnaround of an organization already too far behind in a transforming industry. In the CEO's scathing answers to the board's questions, he used the metaphor of being stuck on a burning oil platform in the middle of the North Sea to describe the position of Nokia's technology platform. He explained they had the choice between going up in flames with the platform or jumping from the thirty-foot-high platform into freezing water. He chose to jump. This metaphor brought a reprimand from the board, even though it was correct. What a way to start as CEO. Transformation was not possible. In the end, Microsoft acquired Nokia. The Nokia CEO has now returned to Microsoft.

"Needed" Questions

Gus Hunt, the former chief technology officer for the CIA, commented in a recent conversation,[3] "Leaders must move from asking the questions they *want* to ask to asking the questions they *need* to ask." In his work with the CIA, the ability to provide information about how the world really worked was critical. Many of his colleagues had mental models of the world based on their past successes and beliefs, sometimes dating back to the Cold War.

It is not only hostile countries that are threatening our security but also loosely coordinated groups of individuals who operate outside any national boundary. The principles of espionage and information acquisition have radically changed. Many leaders who had achieved success during earlier times had mental models based on that prior success; they saw events happening but had not changed their mental models for their work. Gus Hunt's ability to produce information that would change those beliefs was crucial to our national security. In a similar way, the ability of healthcare leaders to ask the questions they need to ask, rather than the ones they want to ask, will ensure the success of their healthcare systems.

Leaders develop a personal style of inquiry. There are a number of ways to get at the same endpoint. In Peter Senge's work on systems thinking[4] these incisive questions are called "wicked questions" because they are precise, they get to the core of the issue, and they expose our assumptions and challenge us.

Open-ended questions are useful. They can begin with; "What if?" or "I know we can't, but if we could, how would we?" The classic line of questioning asks "Why?" Then it asks "Why?" again and again. The questioner may feel like an annoying four-year-old, but the intent is to drill down on assumptions.

Healthcare leaders are experts in their field. Neuropsychological research shows that, as we receive information, it is immediately categorized and made to fit into mental models developed in the course of becoming experts.[5] Most of the time, the efficiency created by filing input into a pre-existing model is a huge benefit. The problem occurs when the situation is changing. Leaders may be filing new information into old mental models. The CIA and Nokia are prime examples of something we all do, which is to focus on the things that fit into our existing models of the world.

Let's test ourselves. Look around the room you are in right now. Identify everything in the room that is blue. Make a note of all of the blue items, and really notice them: where are they, how big are they, what color of blue are they? Now close your eyes and re-create the scene. Your test is to recall all the yellow items. You retain what you focus on. You start with your mental model of a "blue focus," then the world changes to a yellow focus. Incisive questioning, particularly with a diverse group, allows you to have enough lenses that you can see most of the "colors" in a situation.

If you have not already, watch the original video on YouTube of the world-famous selective attention test from Daniel Simons and Christopher Chabris.* This is the test where you count the number of times people pass a ball to each other—and something happens. When people are focused, such as when they are trying very hard to keep up with day-to-day work, they can miss the big things. Developing the practice of questioning with your team, particularly of asking incisive questions, can help point to the unexpected big things.

It is important not only to practice incisive questioning with your team, but to encourage outside organizations to ask questions from their perspective. It is also valuable for you to ask them questions. Your questions may be about their organization's transformation by digitization and disruptive scientific innovation. They may have helpful insights into serving n = 1.

Customers, n = 1 individuals, are particularly important, as they will have a perspective on their healthcare experience. Many organizations find that including their high-potential, up-and-coming leaders in inquiry sessions is an excellent developmental process. The future depends on serving n = 1. The high-potential leaders on your team must build mental models that correspond to that future.

Questions beget thinking. Thinking creates our mental models. Our mental models determine how we process information and how we create the future. The art of skillful questioning is a foundation of transformative change.

* https://www.youtube.com/watch?v=vJG698U2Mvo

Chapter 1. Questions:

- What is your organizational culture regarding incisive questions?

- Are questions important to your organization? Why?

- How do you, as a leader, feel about questioning?

- Do you practice asking questions?

PART II

The Unstoppable Forces
of n = 1

ncisive questioning skills must be applied to develop a deep understanding of the environmental forces impacting healthcare. What does the power of n = 1, the unique individual, really mean for our organization? How will other transformative forces change us? Many times the magnitude and amount of change creates a sense of organizational chaos. Leaders must bring understanding to the seemingly chaotic change. They must create conceptual frameworks to communicate and execute necessary change. What follows are frameworks and questions to stimulate that leadership process.

CHAPTER 2

The Social Context for the Forces of Transformation

This book's framework for transformation is: n = 1. The uniqueness of each individual is transforming healthcare.

The two key elements influencing healthcare are transformative forces and their social context. Transformative forces are digitization and disruptive scientific innovation, which are global and which impact every part of our lives. The social context includes risk transference and sacred trust. These are part of the social context unique to healthcare.

Transformative forces act on individuals and healthcare within the framework of the social context. There are two key elements in social context: the unsustainable cost of healthcare, which results in transference of risk, and the sacred trust of the healing relationship between patient and clinician.

Forces will change the expectations and behaviors of individuals, the n = 1, within this context. The leader's role is to connect the dots between these forces: the social context and the necessary competencies of her organization.

While it's helpful to learn from transformation in other industries, healthcare is different. Healthcare's social context is unlike that of other industries. The business model of insurance-based fee-for-service payment is unique. Transference of economic risk from employers and governments to individuals is transforming healthcare's business models. Altered incentives and payment models create context for the forces of transformation for both the individual and the health system. This will be discussed in more depth later.

Healthcare is not just a business. Healthcare is a profession, a calling, and a sacred trust. The professionalism of clinicians and their commitment to patients is an important context that influences the individual as well as the healthcare organization.

How transformation impacts healthcare organizations is profoundly influenced by the social context, just as the importance of a liver, kidney, or heart cannot be fully appreciated without understanding its connection the functioning of the entire body. The forces must be understood, but their full implication requires the social context.

This book will not provide a detailed analysis of whether healthcare costs are too high. There is an assumption that the costs are increasing at an unsustainable rate. There is ample documentation and discussion of this fact elsewhere. This unsustainable trend and cost will create a market context that will influence the transformation of healthcare.

Transferring Financial Risk

The primary holders of healthcare insurance risk are governments and employers. There are approximately 165 million individuals covered by employer health benefit programs and other private coverage, 46 million covered by Medicare, 51 million by Medicaid programs, 8 million by private exchanges, and 48 million uninsured. These numbers are approximate as they are continuously shifting, and these categories are highly summarized.

The United States government has all or partial responsibility for the 97 million individuals covered by Medicare and Medicaid, as well as the obligations of Social Security, in addition to those covered by the Department of Defense and the Department of Veterans Affairs. The majority of the expenditures of the government are in insurance and military, as noted in Figure 1. It is no wonder that economist Paul Krugman described the federal government as "an insurance company with an army."

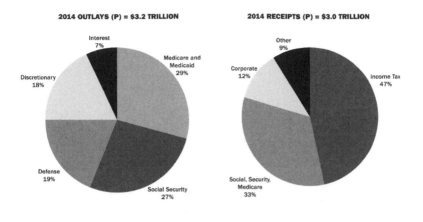

Figure 1. 2014 U.S. Governmental Outlays and Receipts (projected)
Source: The Health Management Academy Research; Congressional Budget Office.

Health insurance costs have been increasing dramatically, and the actuarial risks of these insurance programs make them difficult to predict. The only thing worse than cost escalation is uncertainty. As healthcare utilization and costs increase, insurers and employers are seeking ways to minimize their risk exposure. Figure 1 shows the breakdown of U.S. Federal outlays.

There are a number of healthcare cost containment strategies being implemented by those holding risk: benefit reduction, narrowing networks, reduced reimbursement, and increased regulation, among others. One approach, which provides predictability and potential for cost management, is to transfer risk to providers and consumers (n = 1). If you can't manage the risk, move it to someone else who can.

In its purest form, fee-for-service payment holds neither the patient nor the provider at risk for the cost or quality of the care. As costs have escalated, there have been incremental refinements to benefits and reimbursement models. The thesis of this book is that more profound change is required.

Risk transference has been increasing over the last twenty-five years, but its pace has accelerated over the last ten years. Response by payers has been to transfer risk to individuals through mechanisms like high-deductible health plans, and to providers through payment models such as DRGs or bundled payment. Risk transference will continue to accelerate and influence transformation.

The underlying principle of risk transfer is that providers and consumers will manage healthcare costs more effectively if they have more responsibility for them. This risk transference addresses moral hazard, which is a core principle of insurance and economics. Basically, it says that an entity may expose itself to more risk if it is not sensitive to the costs caused by that risk. People are generally not sensitive to the costs of their healthcare. Providers are generally not incented for the cost effectiveness of the healthcare utilization they generate.

When risk is transferred to the n = 1, a more retail healthcare system results. The n = 1 is now increasingly at risk for her own money. She is informed and incented to be a better healthcare consumer. The more thoughtful retail purchasing of healthcare may lower costs and trends. Many entrepreneurs and innovators are creating tools to assist these informed consumers. The growth of this retail market, especially that driven by employer-sponsored insurance, is strong.

Choice and control are very important to the n = 1. A consumer is more willing to accept a reduction in her health benefit, thus increasing her risk, if she has a choice in how that benefit is reduced. She will manage her risk by choosing the parameters of coverage, including benefits, network, premium, and deductible. Research by Accenture, presented in Figure 2, shows that 25 percent of employees will choose lower-priced and less-comprehensive coverage as a trade-off for income or other benefits. These trade-offs are weighed against the premium reduction or other gain the employee anticipates.

HEALTH INSURANCE BENEFIT TRADEOFF "LEVER"	% OF SURVEY RESPONDENTS WILLING TO ACCEPT TRADEOFF FOR REDUCED MONTHLY PREMIUM
Higher Deductible	78%
Wellness Program Participation	75%
Less Network Flexibility	26%
Fewer Services Covered	25%
Greater Cost Sharing (e.g., Copay)	23%

Figure 2. Purchasing Behavior. The Benefit Tradeoff: One in four employees will select lower-priced and less-comprehensive coverage as a tradeoff for income and other benefits
Source: Accenture Health Research, 2013.

The highest proportion of employees, as noted in Figure 2, will choose a high-deductible plan. Deductible options in the $2,000–5,000 range are currently the norm. How n = 1 manages this significant amount of money will alter healthcare in the next several years. This is retail healthcare, and it is growing.

The n = 1 risk is limited in this model to the cost of the deductible. The cost of a significant illness will exceed the deductible. Therefore, there will be a network linkage to providers to manage the cost in excess of the deductible. Providers will be at risk for costs above the deductible.

When risk for a group of people is transferred to the provider, a population-based healthcare system results. In the fullest expression of population healthcare, providers assume risk for all healthcare needs of a population over time. They are paid ahead of time for the actuarially determined cost of the care. Providers can also assume risk for a specific chronic disease, episode of illness, or other discrete measurable healthcare event. Narrower risk-management goals may be on a patient-by-patient basis. The goal for the providers is to manage the overall cost of care and provide quality services within the payment received.

Understanding the n = 1, the unique individual, is of paramount importance within population healthcare. Providers must understand the individuals within a population as well as a population as a whole. As we will see, organizations that excel at population-based healthcare also excel at understanding each unique individual.

These two broad categories of risk transference are growing as fee-for-service declines. The transition from decades of fee-for-service incentives to various forms of risk transference is creating a turbulent market. Permutations and blurring of the two basic strategies of risk transference will be the norm. Innovation is evolving in the management of risk transference.

One of the challenges for health systems is that the transition from fee-for-service will not be swift or uniform. In addition, new payment models will likely have many permutations of risk transference. This will create challenges. The business model challenges will be addressed later in the book, as will a deeper look at the impact on the n = 1 of the transference of risk.

The transformative forces of digitization and disruptive scientific innovation will impact healthcare in this societal context of risk-transference and payment-model change. The transformative forces will enable the risk to be transferred to the individual and provider. Successful healthcare organizations, insurers, and individuals will use the forces to successfully manage risk.

After decades of fee-for-service payment, the significant transference of risk is relatively new. The other societal context for the transformational environment is not new; it's as old as medicine. It's what sets healthcare apart from all the other industries that have undergone transformation. It is the core of healthcare and must be preserved.

The Sacred Trust

Physicians and other healthcare professionals have always been skeptical of change. Their concern is, "Will change actually improve things for my patient?" or "Will it potentially do them harm?" The core credo of physicians is, "First do no harm."

The forces of digitization and disruptive scientific innovation, just as in other industries, is transforming healthcare. However, there is a fundamental difference between healthcare and other industries. Healthcare is healing. Healthcare reflects a sacred trust between healthcare professionals and patients.

Healing is more than a diagnosis, treatment protocol, or probabilistic algorithm. Healing is more than a business. Healthcare delivery doesn't occur in a laboratory under ideal circumstances; it takes place in the real world. Patients are frequently frightened, emotional, and uninformed. The sacred trust is the glue that holds a healing relationship together.

The sacred trust integral to a healing relationship is the result of the beliefs of the caregiver and the patient. The essential ingredient is the clinician's absolute commitment to the patient to alleviate disease and suffering. Legal, ethical, and cultural responsibilities for this clinician–patient relationship are defined by society.

Patients, n = 1, at their most vulnerable, open themselves to clinicians. They engage in a dependent relationship that exists in few other places in society. They disclose things. They open themselves to invasive physical treatments. They trust, hope, and believe. Sacred trust is necessary for the healing relationship to occur. Different cultures and beliefs have unique elements of the sacred trust, but it is present in all healing relationships.

What is the potential impact of the transformational forces on the sacred trust? Should clinicians be concerned and skeptical? Transformational forces can potentially damage the healing relationship between the patient and caregiver. For example, digitization, improperly structured, can create a barrier to the interaction between patient and clinician. Perhaps retail-reimbursement models could create a purely transactional relationship between patient and health professional. In some scenarios, payment to providers for population health or bundled payment may create consumer suspicion of provider motives, as the provider might benefit by using less care for patients.

Our mental models for healing relationships will be altered by the transformational forces. The current mental models are of healers as successful experts. These are the same types of mental models we noted in the discussion of experts in the CIA and at Nokia. Things are changing, and the mental models of healthcare must evolve.

The traditional mental model of a physician is a compassionate, all-knowing healer. In this traditional model, the patient comes to the healing relationship vulnerable and dependent. The clinician wields the control and information. The patient is a passive, obedient recipient of the care. This conceptual model, which has been evolving for some time, is still popular on television dramas.

What will take its place? What will become of the sacred trust between clinician and patient?

Some envision the future model for medicine as based solely on algorithms that provide a treatment plan drawing on the latest clinical evidence, which is gleaned from a massive database. The application of the medical knowledge requires no human healing interaction, only analytics. There is value to elements of this mental model, but it will not satisfy the needs of most people faced with important personal health decisions. It misses the human elements of healing, caring, and compassion. It lacks intuition and judgment.

The practice of medicine is both art and science. There must be sacred trust in a healing relationship as well as science.

Transformative forces provide the opportunity for the physician and the patient to have the best possible information within a healing relationship. The transformative forces must serve this relationship, not diminish it.

The future will bring challenges to the sacred trust within the healing relationship, and leaders must remain vigilant to preserve it. The concept of n = 1 is tightly integrated into the personal and human aspects of a healing relationship. Individuals, n = 1, want to be treated in unique, sensitive ways. Most people want a human connection in their care.

Healthcare leaders must create frameworks and mental models demonstrating how the transformative forces enhance the healing relationship, and they must do so explicitly and convincingly. Clinicians should understand change in the context of how care will improve for patients and for their ability to do their work.

Can digitization allow the clinician to know the patient even better? Will disruptive scientific innovation allow a more individualized therapeutic relationship? Will the patient know more about the clinician? Can they know more about their healthcare problems and potential solutions? The sacred trust in the healing relationship has always been unique and individual. Can the transformative forces deepen that relationship?

How will digitization and disruptive scientific innovation make the healing relationship stronger? Will clinicians and patients have information at their fingertips and spend more time on the healing relationship? Many physicians are engaging in joint decision-making with the n = 1. The movement to partnership-based healing relationships is well established. The focus of the n = 1 transformation will be on the further evolution of these relationships, using the transformative forces of digitization and disruptive scientific innovation.

There are many examples of digitization enhancing the relationship between non-healthcare service providers and customers. The sacred trust of the healing relationship is different from an Enterprise car rental return or USAA call center interaction. These companies provide a deeper individualized connection with a customer, aided by digitization. This enhances the experience of the n = 1. Where have you experienced similar connections between digitization and personal service? What do you think the customer experience in these companies will be like in three years?

These elements of societal context influence how digitization and disruptive scientific innovation will impact healthcare. Leaders must have a framework for these forces and how they may impact their organizations. They do not need to be experts in genomics, engineering, or computer science, but they should have knowledge of how these forces are evolving and how they may impact healthcare.

Leaders of the transformative forces, such as computational biology, cloud computing, predictive analytics, genomics, microbiomes, and others, unanimously believe that we are just at the beginning of a massive shift in the way we think about our field and that our understanding of the field is different than it was five years ago. Everything is changing as digitization and scientific innovation rapidly transform our field.

Healthcare leaders must connect the dots between these rapidly changing forces to their organizations, all within the societal context of healthcare.

Chapter 2. Social Context:

• Are you clear with yourself about your mental models, beliefs, and orthodoxies about healthcare? Can you be explicit about what they are?

• What happens if the sacred trust in the healing relationship is no longer important in healthcare?

• When risk is transferred to consumers, what will be their expectations of your organization? What are your three priorities to address that?

CHAPTER 3

Digitization

Digitization refers to the conversion of information from analog to digital form. In digital form, information is analyzed, stored, and communicated. Digitization, within decades, has changed every element of our lives. However, widespread digitization in healthcare is relatively new.

The world is now based in zeros and ones. Our lives have been digitalized. The conversion from an analogue to a digital world has been profound and has changed the behaviors and expectations of individuals throughout the world.

People think based on their mental model of the world. A mental model is an internal representation of reality, a selected set of concepts and their relationships. Based on the individual's experiences, they are then used to understand reality and the environment. We previously discussed the mental models of leaders, based on their past experiences and expertise. Their mental models for their companies changed as their businesses changed. Pervasive digitization has changed the mental models of individuals throughout the world. Through these changes, digitization has created the $n = 1$, unique individuals.

These mental models create expectations and beliefs. The $n = 1$ expects ease of access to information. He also expects little difficulty in completing transactions in everything from retail to banking to filling up with gas. He expects options and choices based on his preferences. He expects the devices in his world to be communicating with each other to make his life easier.

Smartphone technology has allowed the n = 1 to carry the majority of the knowledge of the world in his pocket, something that was unthinkable just over a decade ago. The expectation of this democratization of information is changing political systems and challenging governments. The democratization of information is not about information solely created and organized by experts. Twitter, Facebook, and Wikipedia organize information gathered and shared by the n = 1.

The free access to information has emboldened the decision-making of the n = 1. Information customized to his preferences leads to informed decision-making. He expects his decisions to be implemented flawlessly.

The consequences of digitization have not been without controversy. The beliefs and concerns of individuals regarding privacy challenge digitization and the use of information. These concerns may modify digitization, but they will not stop it.

The incredible power that digitization has brought individuals has changed their expectations of how things should work. Thus the term, n = 1, for individuals with these expectations. The mental models of individuals are further modified by disruptive scientific innovation. The impact of these forces on people occurs within the social context of risk transference and are dramatically changing the n = 1 interaction with healthcare.

To be clear, digitization doesn't just provide tools and insights; it fundamentally changes the individual's expectations and his mental models of the world. The continued advancement of digitization will further increase the n = 1 expectations.

Healthcare is in the early stages of digitization. There are many reasons why it has not moved faster; among other things, it's a highly fragmented cottage industry, with little sensitivity to cost and with skepticism among clinicians about change.

The mental models of healthcare professionals are important. Their internal representations of reality have been built by decades of success as experts. These can include mental models of how patient information is shared with clinicians, how the information from diagnostic studies is shared, or any other aspect of healthcare. Models that have worked extremely well in the past are retained. The mental models regarding knowledge and information in healthcare become its "information architecture." These mental models of information can have roots in earlier times in medicine.

Thirty years ago, a young internist began his medical practice. His office consisted of another physician, nurses, and support staff. The medical practice was paper-based, including prescriptions, laboratory tests, and the patient's chart. Physicians "handed off" patients to the physician on call, using 3" x 5" note cards to convey information; these would then be given to the office manager for billing. The latest medical knowledge came from a few sources: *The New England Journal of Medicine*, regular specialty conferences, and, of course, visits from pharmaceutical representatives.

Medical records and other data were kept on paper files in huge cabinets that were constantly being exchanged between the file clerks, coders, billing experts, and clinical staff. Information was filed chronologically, but finding records was a challenge at times and could not always be retrieved when needed. Other than a manual problem list, there was not much synthesis of the patient's information in his chart—information meant to provide the basis for clinical decision-making. If an on-call physician cared for a partner's patient after office hours, lack of information could pose problems.

This scenario is from a long time ago, but for some it is just beginning to change. A decade or so later, analytics were beginning to be used in the HMO world. The chief medical officer for a health plan was reviewing the practice patterns of physicians in a small local community. He identified a pattern of inappropriate, high-cost antibiotic use for outpatient infections. The CMO had claims data specific for each patient and physician. He met with local physicians and shared with them the unattributed data of their antibiotic use. This was then compared to the use patterns of statewide physicians. The CMO asked what was different about their patients. There was silence. Finally, the physician who was the leading prescriber of this antibiotic said, "The pharmaceutical rep said all of you were prescribing this antibiotic because you are all convinced of its effectiveness in all these conditions."

These were all excellent physicians trying to do their best job for their patients. This was the first time they had information and analytics to guide their outpatient care. They appreciated the information from the health plan and were anxious for more because more robust information architecture would help their patients. What was their mental model of information to improve clinical practice? They treated small numbers of patients and often had only anecdotal outcome information. Access to a more comprehensive information architecture was valuable. It was critical the information was presented in the right way.

Digitization's impact on the information architecture for physicians has been slow to progress. Some specialties in medicine, such as thoracic surgeons, anesthesiologists, and neonatal intensivists, have collected and analyzed data for some time, but this has not been widespread across all specialties. However, over the last decade, digitization has increased. Many diagnostic and therapeutic modalities are highly digitized and automated. Each of these individual modalities generates significant information through digitization.

Young clinicians familiar with digitization have been innovators within healthcare. Computer-savvy physicians have been responsible for many of the changes that are moving digitization forward. In many cases, they see the need because they are very comfortable in the digital world. They are the n = 1 of clinicians, and they expect digitalization to work for them in patient care. They have an understanding of what it can do and the initiative to make it happen.

The automation of the electronic health record (EHR) is big step. According to a report in *Health Affairs* noted in Figure 3, the use of EHRs by physicians has increased steadily from 2004 to 2013, due in part to funding from the federal government's HITECH program, passed in 2009. According to the Centers for Disease Control and Prevention, by 2012 more than 50 percent of eligible professionals (mostly physicians) had demonstrated meaningful use and received an incentive payment from the federal HITECH program.

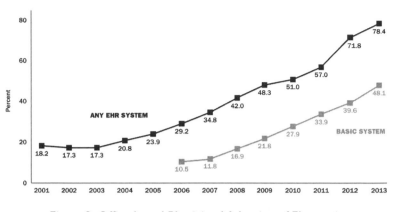

**Figure 3. Office-based Physicians' Adoption of Electronic
Health Record Systems, 2001–2013[6]**

Source: CDC/NCHS, National Ambulatory Medical Care Survey, 2001–2012.

For hospitals, a similar pattern of growth occurred. A *Health Affairs* article reported, as noted in Figure 4, that in 2008 just 9 percent of hospitals had adopted EHR's, but by 2013, approximately 60 percent had demonstrated meaningful use of the EHR. That is remarkable growth.

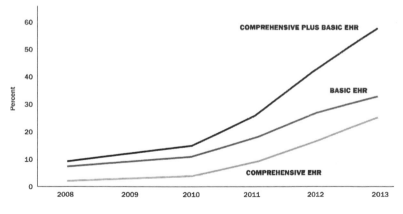

**Figure 4. Hospitals' Adoption of Electronic
Health Record Systems, 2008–2013[7]**

Source: Adler-Milstein et al. "More Than Half of US Hospitals Have At Least A Basic
EHR, But Stage 2 Criteria Remains Challenging For Most." *Health Affairs*, 2014.
Authors' analysis of data from the American Hospital Association Annual Survey–IT
Supplements, 2008–13. Note: Data are weighted to adjust for nonrespondents bias based
on observed differences between survey respondents and nonrepsondents.

Implementation of EHR is expensive, risky, and resource-intensive. The return on investment is uncertain. So what motivated so many organizations to take on the challenge? The federal government created incentives for adoption of digital health records as part of the stimulus package. This was the push that was necessary to move digitization of healthcare. These "meaningful use" incentives for automation motivated most healthcare organizations. In addition, more effective billing and potential for streamlining administrative processes provided an economic rationale.

The EHR strategies were based on current business models, rather than anticipating the digital future. This is understandable, as this is a big step for health systems. The EHR systems, for the most part, are decades old and were designed to capture the transactional nature of medical practice. This is major progress, but it is important to recognize the rationale.

So where is digitization in healthcare organizations going? With the EHR implemented in the vast majority of provider organizations, what's the vision? What should the information architecture be for the future of the healthcare organization?

Creating an Information Architecture

Earlier, we discussed the information architecture of thirty years ago. What is the evolution of healthcare to meet the needs of n = 1? What is the vision for this new information architecture? Change can be so profound that it's difficult for leaders to see. Digitization has changed the fabric of the world and the expectations and behaviors of individuals, n = 1. How must the healthcare organization be transformed by digitization to meet those expectations of the n = 1?

Discussions with healthcare leaders bring to the surface similar ideas regarding the components of an information architecture. They describe an incremental flow to the development of the architecture.

These are the common steps:

- Shared vision for digitization
- Development of clinical and administrative leading practices
- Standardization of clinical and administrative processes
- Data capture, analysis, and use
- Predictive analytics
- Enabling individualized medicine for the n = 1

This information architecture will be customized by every organization. Most organizations have progressed in all these areas. The framework makes it helpful to see the connections. Digitization supports the overall strategy of the organization and is not the strategy.

These discussions with leaders suggest frameworks are loosely in place in most organizations, but they may not have understanding or agreement across leadership. The stress and the challenges of implementing EHRs have been all-consuming.

Shared Vision for Information Architecture

The diversity of healthcare organizations and their missions will create a diversity of visions for information architecture. This is where the incisive questions of leaders will shape the organizational vision. The specifics of the vision are less important than the process to reach the vision. It is most important that the vision is shared and understood. Leaders must be looking over the horizon to see the possibilities of rapidly moving information science.

Development of Leading Practices

Organizations must identify the best ways to do things before they automate. Healthcare organizations come from a heritage of profound variation in clinical and administrative practice. Much like our example of the physicians prescribing antibiotics earlier, the origin of practices is often obscure or anecdotal.

Organizations that automate their historic less-than-optimal patient care and productivity processes are "paving the cow paths." Gaining agreement to utilizing leading practices prior to digitization is necessary to assure clinical and administrative improvement. These are extraordinarily challenging discussions, as clinicians and management have their own ideas about what is best. This is also a never-ending commitment.

The movement over the last decade or so toward leading practices in healthcare has exposed the variation in medical practice, and this must be addressed within the digitization process. It arises from many different sources. For example, only 20 percent of medical treatments are "proven" through rigorous scientific methods. This lack of proof has many understandable causes, such as difficulty in conducting double-blind studies and some treatment modalities, such as surgical procedures; long time frames to assess results; and ethical considerations about withholding care. In other words, scientific proof can be elusive for many good reasons[8]:

- Because of each patient's unique biologic nature, even a "proven" treatment is just a statement of probability for the success of that treatment for a given individual.
- Individual value systems and beliefs are at play for both the patient and the physician. They influence care, and they may not comply with the best medical science
- There are large geographic variations in medical practice that are poorly understood, according to the Dartmouth Atlas.
- Physicians utilize familiar care processes that their experience shows will give them the best results, even if those techniques are not leading practices.
- Financial incentives for physician and patient may guide the treatment modality.

For these and other reasons, there can be a difference between the leading practice and the treatment used. The opportunity with digitization is to develop a greater transparency and agreement of what works best.

Standardization of Clinical and Administrative Processes

After leading practices are identified, they must be standardized across all participants within the healthcare organization. Identifying leading practices is hard enough, but the agreement to standardize can be even more difficult. There are innumerable examples of leading practices that are known but not adhered to by some clinicians.

A standardized approach to the administrative and clinical process is necessary to create data that can be used to refine the processes. Without standardization, the data is difficult if not impossible to interpret.

Standardization and subsequent automation of leading practices greatly increases the likelihood of their being used. Standardization must not be rigid in clinical decision-making. There must always be the ability for clinical judgment to prevail, even if it is in conflict with leading practice. What is important is to capture the rationale of the exception and build that into the standards.

The commitment to standardization goes back to the vision for digitization, which is about how to standardize a process so comparable data can be collected to improve it.

Ultimately, the care for the n = 1 is an individualized approach to treatment. In order to have processes in place to individualize, processes must initially be standardized.

Data Capture, Analysis, and Use

The game-changing opportunity for healthcare is the use of data. In the past, data has been "locked" in paper charts or disparate systems. In the last five years, a tsunami of data has flowed into healthcare. The EHR, patient monitoring, and other data-gathering tools have opened the floodgates.

The n = 1 individualized medicine will require sophisticated data and analytics. The standardization and automation required to implement EMR and other systems can make the outcomes of clinical-care processes more visible. Patient information is increasingly gathered, and clinicians are beginning to analyze the differences in approaches to clinical processes in patients. When this analysis is undertaken over vast numbers of patients, and analyzed with sophisticated mathematical capabilities, new insights will result.

All of this would not be possible without the efforts to identify, standardize, and automate leading practices.

There are challenges to the digitization of healthcare. The opportunity to automate care processes in multiple areas of healthcare, such as inpatient, outpatient, laboratory, radiology, and others, has led to the implementation of many different technologies. Interoperability challenges between these technologies place limits on the ability to capture and utilize the data. Leaders understand the importance of resolving these issues.

The user interface between clinicians and many of the digital technologies of patient care are not optimal, and as a result clinicians are faced with lost productivity. The computer screen can become a barrier to the sacred trust of the healing relationship with a patient. As these impediments are resolved, the realization of the vision will be easier. Making interfacing with technology easier will allow clinicians to more fully use the information available.

Predictive Analytics and Machine Learning

Predictive analytics, sometimes marketed as "big data," allows us to use massive amounts of data, from many sources, to identify correlations and trends in that information. When describing big data, terms often used are the velocity, volume, variability, veracity and value of data. This means that the more information of all kinds that is available, the better the ability to find correlations.

The mathematics, physics, computational capability, and understanding of predictive analytics have evolved rapidly in the last several years. Their use in retail, government, and social networking has changed our lives. Familiar and obvious examples include Amazon marketplace recommendations, Facebook data assisting retailers in customizing marketing to the n = 1, and the NSA's capability to pro file virtually anybody, anywhere.

How can we separate the marketing hype of big data from the reality and potential of predictive analytics? How will predictive analytics change healthcare?

Predictive analytics tools access large amounts of data, which in healthcare can include administrative information, laboratory and radiology results, "real time" vital signs, and other patient-specific information. Algorithms are created by data scientists based on the likelihood that certain abnormalities in any set of data could be associated with a disease.

Data scientists, who are at the heart of any predictive analytic program, have honed their ability to understand the problem at hand. They work closely with their clients, who are content experts. Data scientists are frequently statisticians and mathematicians. They ask very different questions than administrative or clinical experts. Data scientists report that getting the content experts to define the problem clearly is often the most difficult part of a project. Once the problem is defined, they then can build the mathematical algorithms and access the data to begin looking for correlations that will be helpful in solving the problem.

The problems can be retrospective, based on existing static databases. What are the factors that might be correlated with a specific disease? They can be real-time, and have data feeding into the algorithm at high velocity from multiple sources. What patients we are currently caring for are at risk for a certain problem? Can we identify them earlier by constantly looking for correlations in multiple different data streams?

Sepsis is an infection that invades the bloodstream, creating severe complications. It has an extraordinarily high mortality rate, causing as many as 48 percent of inpatient deaths in some institutions. Successful treatment depends on early identification and therapeutic intervention.

Providence Health and Services created early warning systems for sepsis, using predictive analytics. Historically, the nursing staff would make rounds to take the vital signs of each patient and assess his condition. If they found the vital signs abnormal or the patient "didn't look good," they might seek another opinion or call the physician. Lab tests may or may not make it back to the patient's bedside in time to help with the decision-making. The ability to synthesize the clinical picture can be a challenge for even the most competent clinicians.

In the predictive analytic model for identifying early sepsis, there are significant tools available to assist the clinicians. In addition to nurses making clinical rounds, data streams from everything associated with the patient go to a central location. This data includes administrative, lab, radiology, vital signs, monitor, and many other data elements. The algorithms analyze this data. If the algorithm determines there are criteria correlated with potential sepsis, clinical staff is automatically alerted electronically by the system. Thus, patients at high risk for sepsis are identified early, and the nursing and clinical staff can focus more resources on them. Providence reduced sepsis mortality by half. A former leader at Amazon, now working with Providence in this area, commented that Amazon uses "recommendation engines," and healthcare providers need recommendation engines, too. These engines guide clinical interactions and decisions.

The current results in sepsis are encouraging, but there is additional promise as the algorithms are continually enhanced and refined. As more data stream into the system, the predictive analytic tools become increasingly sophisticated in the ability not only to spot patients who are in early sepsis, but to identify those who may appear to be developing sepsis but in reality are not. In addition, as more and more data are gathered about sepsis or any other disease, our understanding of the most efficacious treatment modalities is enhanced. The recommendation engines are continually refined so the clinicians closest to the patient have the best information.

Predictive analytics is based on the fact that there is now massive data available, and it is growing faster than we can comprehend. Eric Schmidt, Executive Chairman of Google, observed that humankind generated five exabytes (one quintillion bytes) of data from the dawn of civilization until 2003.[9] We now produce five exabytes of data every two days, and the pace is accelerating. Healthcare is at the beginning of digitization and the generation of patient data. The implementation of systems such as automated EHRs has only just entered a rapid growth of generating enormous quantities of data.

Several years ago, Chris Anderson, the editor of *Wired* magazine, coined the term "the petabyte age."[10] In the article, he described the impact of massive data on decision-making. He described Google's founding philosophy as: "We don't know why this page is better than that one: if the statistics of incoming links say it is, that's good enough. No semantic or causal analysis is required." The collection of massive amounts of information drives their ability to develop correlations.

That philosophy allowed Google to translate languages without actually "knowing" them. Google entered all possible translations of most languages into their database; this included all types of written material, including slang and poor translations. It then developed correlations between the languages with predictive analytics. It did use expert translation skills. The results demonstrate that Google Translate can, given equal corpus data, translate Mandarin into Farsi as easily as it can translate French into German. This is also why it can match ads to content without any knowledge or assumptions about the ads or the content.

Predictive analytics analyzes massive amounts of data with statistical algorithms to produce correlations. These correlations can give insight, and not infrequently the insights are surprising. The correlations in a retail site such as Amazon, where "if you liked this product, you'll like this product," have proven to be highly valued. Have you ever wondered about the algorithm "thinking" that created some of your recommendations?

Data scientists report that the correlations they find are often a surprise to the content experts. The experts often have preconceptions, or mental models, as to the causation or nature of a problem, and when the correlations show something very different, they are skeptical. This is healthy. The success of the use of these tools depends on the partnership and trust of the data scientists and the content expert. This isn't magic; it's statistics.

Automobile insurance companies use massive amounts of information and predictive analytics to determine risk and thus your automobile premium. Auto insurance companies invite you to allow them to install a device to upload your real-time driving information in return for a possibly lower premium. The constantly uploaded data provides high-volume real-time data for risk assessment and claims management.

One rationale for insurers transferring risk was moral hazard. Moral hazard is based in the asymmetry of information between the insurer and the insured; or, to put it differently, it is difficult to predict how behavior changes when people are insured against losses. The insurer doesn't absolutely know the riskiness of the insured's behavior. Predictive analytics can reduce the asymmetry of information. It democratizes the information for the insurer. Additionally, it probably has a sentinel effect on driving habits as well. Does the use of predictive analytics in these ways have potential uses as risk is transferred to providers?

We must remember the old axiom "correlation does not imply causation." That is to say, predictive analytics can identify correlates to a certain problem, but it does not mean that those correlates are causative. This is, at first blush, at variance with the scientific method, which seeks to prove causation. The proof of causation is the basis of medical science. However, even with the scientific method, there is ultimately an assignment of a probability when evaluating the likelihood of an event occurring to an individual person.

Scientific method, which requires large volumes of heterogeneous people to make its conclusions, can only be predictive as to a unique individual's response or condition. As the unique nature of the biology of each individual is clearly delineated, the limits of large-scale population testing will become even more apparent. Drug development and the unique pharmacokinetics of individuals is a prime example. One drug dose is too much and is toxic for some people, and the same dose is too little to be effective for others. Nonetheless, the cultural aspects of using correlation from predictive analytics in patient care may be challenging for clinicians.

According to *Big Data: A Revolution That Will Transform How We Live, Work, and Think*,[11] "In a big data world . . . we won't have to be fixated on causality; instead, we can discover patterns and correlations in the data that offer us novel and invaluable insights. The correlations may not tell us precisely why something is happening, but they alert us to what is happening. And in many situations, this is good enough. If millions of electronic medical records reveal that certain cancer sufferers who take a certain combination of aspirin and orange juice see their disease go into remission, then the exact cause for the remission and health may be less important than the fact that they lived."

The use of predictive analytics may be able to reveal correlations in diseases like MS, autism, and even obesity. Bringing massive amounts of disparate data together increases the likelihood that some correlation, not previously suspected, may be implicated in these diseases. The next chapter will discuss how the increased ability to monitor the $n = 1$ physiology will further increase our understanding of pathology.

The excitement and hype around predictive analytics and big data is tempered by the reality of its early use in healthcare. In "The Parable of Google Flu: Traps in Big Data Analysis" by David Lazer, et al.,[12] the authors show that the predictions made by one of the leading organizations in big data were decidedly inaccurate. Google Flu Trends (GFT), a leading example of health-related big data, uses flu-related search queries to fuel algorithms to predict the circulation of flu in the world. The use of the 500 million Google searches every day fuels the GFT predictions.

The predictions overestimated the prevalence of the flu in the 2011–2012 and 2012–2013 seasons by more than 50 percent. From August 2011 to September 2013, GFT over-predicted the prevalence of flu in 100 out of 108 weeks. If fact, last winter GFT predicted that 11 percent of the U.S. population had the flu, which is much larger than the CDC's actual number of 6 percent.

There were many problems with GFT, as noted by the authors. They included search terms not reflecting incidences of disease, problematic associations in the model, and failure to anticipate unexpected events (like the 2009 H1N1-A pandemic). As Lazer says, "A number of associations in the models were really problematic; it was doomed to fail."

These researchers believe predictive analytics can be more useful if paired with other data-analysis tools they call "small data," the more traditional form of data collection and analysis. The combination of big data, small data, and human interpretation would seem to be the best way to create accurate predictive models. One of the messages from the authors is the need for transparency and collaboration in gathering and utilizing big data. Healthcare leaders may want to consider the limitations and scientific errors Google created through its lack of transparency and cooperation. Transparent and cooperative settings are more likely to harness the power of health data now becoming available.

Big data is not a magical tool that provides the ability to "know all." It is a tool best used with knowledge of its strengths and limitations, and it is strengthened by being paired with experienced, expert humans. It is early in the use of this tool in healthcare. The potential in the next five years, as more data are available and the science of predictive analytics advances, is both exciting and difficult to fully comprehend.

In their book *The Second Machine Age*, Erik Brynjolfsson and Andrew McAfee[13] describe "freestyle" chess tournaments, which offer some insight into healthcare's transformation. The ability for data analytics to transform healthcare will depend on the combination of analytical tools and clinicians' expert intuition and strategic thinking. The freestyle chess tournaments are an example of that combination.

Computers today can beat any grandmaster in a chess match. In "freestyle" events, teams can include any combination of human and digital players. The outcomes have surprised some people, including experts. One of them was Garry Kasparov, the world chess champion from 1986 to 2005. He was defeated in 1997 by the IBM computer Deep Blue in a highly publicized match.

Kasparov observed that, in a 2005 freestyle contest, "The teams of human plus machine dominated even the strongest computers." He went on to explain, "The chess machine Hydra, which is a chess-specific supercomputer like Deep Blue, was no match for a strong human player using a relatively weak laptop. Human strategic guidance combined with the tactical acuity of the computer was overwhelming. The surprise came at the conclusion of the event. The winner was revealed not to be a grandmaster with a state-of-the-art PC, but a pair of amateur American chess players using three computers at the same time. Their skill at manipulating and 'coaching' their computers to look very deeply into positions effectively counteracted the superior chess understanding of their grandmaster opponents and the greater computational power of other participants. Weak amateur + machine + better process was superior to a strong computer alone and, more remarkably, superior to a strong human + machine + inferior process."

Thus, digitization, which is rapidly changing the world, is beginning to change healthcare. From the early days of automation of laboratory and radiographic procedures to the recent ubiquitous implementation of EHRs, digitization and the use of data in healthcare is experiencing exponential growth. This change in the information architecture available to clinicians will require a thoughtful analysis of clinical processes that will likely result in tectonic changes in medical practice. The computational ability to digitize and analyze healthcare is a powerful trend. This trend both supports, and is supported by, another major trend, that of disruptive innovation.

Chapter 3. Digitization:

- Is healthcare different from every other industry that has been changed by digitization? Why?

- What are three ways those differences will influence the impact of digitization?

- What are the top three lessons to be learned from other industries as they were digitized? How can your healthcare organization incorporate those lessons in its strategic plan and budget?

- How will the delivery of healthcare change if patients have similar information as providers?

CHAPTER 4

Disruptive Scientific Innovation

Scientific innovation is occurring at breakneck speed. Because it is changing our fundamental understandings of how things work, much of this innovation is disruptive. This disruptive innovation is impacting healthcare, where our concept of what is possible is changing dramatically. The technological possibilities for healthcare are exploding. Our understanding of human biology is radically being altered, and healthcare leaders must cultivate an understanding of these disruptive scientific innovations.

Healthcare and medicine have historically been innovative; clinicians always want to find the best ways to help their patients. However, disruptive innovations in healthcare have always faced challenges in adoption.

Dr. Barry Marshall's Story

The story of Dr. Barry Marshall and peptic ulcers is an instructive case of disruptive innovation in healthcare.[14] In 1982, Dr. Marshall, an Australian physician, identified a bacterium, *Helicobacter pylori*, in the stomachs of patients with gastritis and ulcers. The medical thinking at the time was that no bacteria could survive in the harsh acidity of the stomach. It's notable that the bacterium had been identified decades earlier, but its significance was discounted and the discovery forgotten. Dr. Marshall observed it in biopsies, but the bacterium was difficult to grow outside of the stomach. In fact, it wasn't grown outside the body until Petri dishes in his lab were accidentally left out for five days over an Easter weekend.

Dr. Marshall and associates published a paper contending that most peptic ulcers and gastritis were caused by this bacterium and not by stress or spicy foods, as had been assumed previously. This was met with skepticism in the medical community. In 1987, to demonstrate the bacterium as the causative organism, Dr. Marshall drank a flask of the culture of the bacteria. Several days later he became ill with nausea and vomiting. Gastritis was demonstrated on endoscopy. A biopsy showed the presence of the bacteria.

Dr. Marshall and his research partner, Dr. Robin Warren, demonstrated that eradicating *H. pylori* with antibiotics had cured the ulcers. In 1994, the U.S. National Institute of Health (NIH) published an opinion stating that the most recurrent duodenal and gastric ulcers are caused by *H. pylori* and recommended antibiotics. Previous therapy for these potentially debilitating and life-threatening ulcers had been antacids, diet changes, and even major surgical procedures that profoundly impacted patients' lives. Even after the NIH published its opinion, it took several additional years for this approach to become standard medical practice.

Dr. Marshall said that during his efforts to prove the nature of this disease, he felt as though, in his words, "everyone was against me." Long-standing beliefs regarding peptic ulcer disease as well as long-established incentives for treatment were barriers to disruptive change. The list of doubters included medical educators, physicians, insurers, pharmaceutical-device manufacturers, hospitals, and others. The spirit of innovation is alive and well, but changing professional opinions takes time and evidence.

As the antibiotic treatment for peptic ulcer disease became commonplace, the incidence of the disease diminished. The new peptic ulcer disease motto was, "The only good *H. pylori* is a dead *H. pylori*." The incidence of *H. pylori* in the GI tract has diminished over the years. There is evidence to suggest a correlation with the lack of *H. pylori* and the development of gastro-esophageal reflux disease, GERD. Research has identified multiple different types of *H. pylori* in humans, some related to disease and some contributing to health. The genetic makeup of each individual also plays a role in her response to the bacteria. This disruptive innovation in treating a serious illness has not proven as straightforward as initially thought. It is one of the first insights into the fascinating and complicated world of the human microbiome.

Dr. Marshall and Dr. Warren were awarded the Nobel Prize in physiology or medicine in 2005 for their discovery of the role of *H. pylori* in gastritis and peptic ulcer disease. Research continues in this area.

Healthcare has traditionally been a fertile source of innovation and challenges to established knowledge. As we have discussed, medicine is both art and science, and clinicians continually seek new ways to provide better patient care. The changes that are occurring in digitization, biology, predictive analytics, and electronics are creating fertile ground for disruptive innovation. In many areas, we are finding that our fundamental understanding of clinical science and human biology is changing rapidly. The ability to measure, communicate, and analyze information is rapidly improving. What will be the impact of disruptive innovation on the healthcare system and on patients?

Advancements in science are contributing to the understanding of the unique individual, n = 1. There are two broad categories of disruptive scientific innovation: technological advancement (including mobile devices, apps, and sensors) and biologic advancement.

Innovation is not invention; it is not a new scientific discovery. Innovation is a "recombination," a merging of existing functions. For example, the first Apple iPod was not an invention. It was a combination of existing technologies that provided a new, customized music service.

There is an explosion of innovation in the technological and biologic areas enabled by digitization. This explosion provides the opportunity to combine technological and biological innovations in what are termed "recombinant innovations." Thus, the advances in technology, physics, and mathematics accelerate the advances in biologic sciences. Fields like computational biology are accelerating our understanding of basic human biology. Healthcare innovation is moving faster than ever, and digitization and recombination are two reasons why that is so.

Technological advancement enabled by digitization continues to move at breakneck speed. Technological change is impacting everyone. The expectations and behaviors of the n = 1 continue to evolve as technological capabilities progress. Enhanced technological capabilities create new opportunities and challenges for the healthcare system and its leaders.

Mobile Devices and Apps

The proliferation of smartphones over the last five years has been a transformational force in its own right. In 2009, there were very few smartphones in use. According to Google, as of January 2012, there were nearly 100 million smartphones in use in the United States and over 1 billion in use in the world. Mary Meeker, in her 2014 Internet Trends Report, referenced 1.6 billion smartphones in use in the world.[15] This explosive adoption is expected to continue, as only about 30 percent of the world's population currently uses a smartphone. The power of these devices is transformative, and their computing ability and other features will enable consumers to use health services when and where they prefer.

Nearly 90 percent of the U.S. population has the Internet at their fingertips, compared to approximately 95 percent for Iceland, Norway, Sweden, and Denmark. This not only gives consumers the ability to communicate with almost anyone else in the world, but also gives them access to unlimited information, which has revolutionized society, including healthcare.

These devices are not only our phones, communication devices, and web browsers; they are also cameras, GPS devices, and gravimeters. As the price point continues to drop, they will become even more ubiquitous and integrated into daily life, and competition will provide them with even more functionality.

Smartphones and related tools will be an important platform for future healthcare. The power and capabilities of the n = 1 with mobile devices will grow and develop beyond our imagination.

According to *Business Week*,[16] there were 97,000 mobile health applications available for download at major app stores. *Business Week* predicts that the mobile-health-app market may reach $26 billion by 2017. There is intense competition to put healthcare on mobile devices.

The U.S. Federal Drug Administration (FDA) has been struggling with how to appropriately regulate healthcare apps. This has created tension between the technology industry and the medical regulatory infrastructure. As the tech industry finds ways to develop apps that allow individuals to measure, test, and diagnose themselves, the FDA is establishing the role of government regulation. The world of government healthcare regulation is testing the patience of the tech community.

Recently completed FDA guidelines require apps that diagnose or treat conditions to meet similar quality standards as heart stents, ultrasound machines, and other medical devices that can compromise the health of patients if they do not work properly. For such products, the agency requires a 510(K) application, which is the least stringent of the device-approval pathways and does not typically require clinical trials. It is reasonable to expect much more activity from regulators in these areas in the future.

While it is clear that healthcare apps on personal mobile devices will be a therapeutic modality of prime importance in the future, the groundwork is still being laid.

The diversity of those 97,000 apps is remarkable. They fall into several categories:

- *Health measurements* such as Nike's Fuel Band, Fitbit, Withings scale, and blood pressure. Apps measure exercise, stress, nutrition, sleep, weight, and many other aspects of daily life. The apps report information back to the user in various formats, allowing her to improve her health by behavioral change. They do not provide either a diagnosis or treatment.

- *Access to medical records.* Apps like My Chart allow the patient to view her medical records and communicate with a provider. Transparency and patient knowledge are enhanced.

- *Diagnostic capabilities.* This very diverse group of apps, used with the supervision of a provider, includes functions that will measure movements of patients with Parkinson's disease; use GPS to monitor the movements of patients during physical therapy or of people with Alzheimer's; and perform asthma, urine, and blood tests using sensors plugged into the smartphone. One device even allows a provider to remotely view a child's tympanic membranes.

- *Advanced diagnostic and therapeutic capabilities.* When paired with a smartphone advanced sensors are capable of cardiac monitoring, blood oxygenation, and many other key indicators. As sensors become increasingly sophisticated, one can envision apps measuring hundreds of different data points and providing real-time feedback to patient and provider. Remote information-gathering and clinical intervention will transform medicine.

This connectivity of apps to provider intervention is in its infancy, but mobile devices and apps are rapidly increasing in sophistication. Just as smartphones were virtually unknown in 2009, the healthcare applications that will be in use five years from now would sound like science fiction today. What is important to leaders is to understand how rapidly this platform is developing and how to use it to benefit the n = 1.

Although the measurement of exercise and similar uses is interesting and may assist in self-improvement, the real value will lie in the interpretation of data that translates back into therapeutic interventions. A provider guides these interventions. Patients will expect more of apps than just documentation of how they're doing; they want to know "so now what am I supposed to do?"

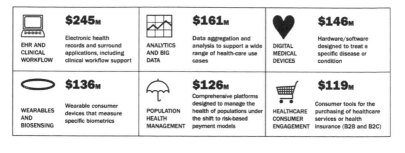

**Figure 5. The Distribution of Capital in Healthcare
Information Innovation in 2013[17]**
Source: Rock Health 2014.

How are health systems identifying ways to connect with n = 1 with apps and provide the value added feedback to the measurements? The adoption of mobile technologies with all their tools and apps has been rapid and profound, and the n = 1 has expectations for using them in most areas of her life. Healthcare providers are being challenged with how their care processes incorporate these technologies. In general, it is younger physicians who tend to adopt these technologies readily and even design their own apps to improve patient care and communicate with their colleagues. For instance, texting has changed the way physicians communicate with each other and with their patients. The ability to include photographs and other content is changing how healthcare is delivered for certain demographics of providers and patients. The boundaries of healthcare become less rigid as communication becomes more mobile.

Demographic differences in technology adoption of all types by younger providers and patients will have a profound impact on the transformation of healthcare. The use of mobile devices and the tools associated with them are becoming second nature; this is how they expect to practice medicine. As they assume leadership of healthcare, there will be a quantum shift in how these tools are applied and used. Forward-looking health systems are engaging younger clinicians and patients to assist them in using these tools more effectively. Healthcare leaders are creating health systems for the future of these clinicians.

Sensors and Monitors

Advances in electrical engineering, physics, communications, and biotechnology allow measurement of health information in radically different ways. Miniature sensors with sophisticated capabilities identify trends and abnormalities in human biochemical composition. There are sensors designed for implantation in the body that can identify cancer proteins in the bloodstream. An individual who had previously been treated for cancer could receive a real-time early warning as to potential recurrence. At the other end of the healthcare spectrum, inexpensive disposable sensors embedded in clothing can monitor the heart rate, respirations, body position, and wakefulness of a baby in the crib.

The noted entrepreneur Vinod Khosla, cofounder of Sun Microsystems and leader of one of the most active firms investing in new healthcare technology and tools, believes that robotics, sensor networks, and complex algorithmic tools that interpret the mountain of data are the future of healthcare.[18] He has said, "Inventors will need to come up with the tools to manage a vast number of data points about each person every day and turn this into useful information and alerts. We will have millions of times more data about patients; we could use this data to prevent disease." He points out that cell phones have dozens of sensors, your car has hundreds of sensors, but the human body has none—and that is going to change.

It is clear that monitors and sensors providing real-time data, coupled with mobile technology and massive computational capabilities, will be game-changers. Devices connected to other devices are called "the Internet of Everything." This supports the goals of the unique individual, n = 1. Sensors collect, mobile devices communicate, and algorithms correlate the data about her status, and personalized medicine will be possible with a specificity never before imagined. The recent rate of adoption of mobile technology indicates that these functions might be standard and more deeply impactful sooner than one might think.

Among physicians today, there is interest about sensors and

monitors but also uncertainty. Many physicians who have patients sending them random blood pressure, weight, and other measurements in an ad hoc fashion aren't sure what to do with the information; nor are patients sure what they should expect from physicians. Clearly, there is an educational aspect to the use of sensors and clinical communication. What is certain is that there are opportunities for innovators and providers to close the loop between measurement and action. The providers and health systems that redefine this connectivity will be in a competitive position.

Many studies have found that, in the treatment of chronic illnesses such as congestive heart failure, asthma, and diabetes, ongoing measurements and interactions between patient and provider can lead to improved outcomes and lower costs. Without a question, as incentives continue to change for reimbursement for both physician and patient, the innovation, adoption, and use of advanced sensors and monitors will increase dramatically.

The New Age of Biology

The last decade has seen the development of dramatic insights into the basic understanding of the biologic sciences. The rapidly deepening understanding of genetics and protein chemistry has led science in directions different than anticipated a decade ago. These have in turn led to insights about how the human body works, even what actually composes the human body. The seemingly clear-cut mechanisms of DNA and its replication turned out to be anything but clear-cut. The importance of proteins, RNA, and other subcellular mechanisms to the understanding of human biology has come to the fore.

A prime example of one of the new understandings of human biology is the human microbiome. Its implications are significant.

Appreciation of the human microbiome is recent, as it is one of the unintended consequences of the Human Genome Project.[19] The Human Microbiome Project,[20] which is similar to the Human

Genome Project, involved 200 scientists at eighty institutions who analyzed the complete bacterial population of hundreds of people. The human body carries roughly ten pounds of bacteria. Measured by genetic material, our body is only 10 percent human and 90 percent bacterial genome. The identification of resident bacteria in every area of our body has been made possible by the rapid gene-sequencing tools developed during the human genome project. The vast majority of these bacteria do not grow outside the human body and can be identified only through genetic sequencing tools.

Bacteria in the gut, skin, mouth, vagina, and other areas of the body have been identified, and patterns of species of bacteria have been determined. However, these patterns of bacterial prevalence vary from person to person and also with time. Work is moving rapidly to determine the impact of this massive amount of resident bacteria and its relation to the human body.

Our microbiome lives with us in a mutually beneficial way. It contributes to our health, and we support its existence. Disturbances in the microbiome can lead to human illness, and changes in it from antibiotics or diet may have a role in disease.

Already it's clear that there are some disorders that directly relate to disturbances to our microbiome. Pseudomembranous colitis is caused by an overgrowth of the bacteria *C. difficile*, which overgrows in the intestinal tract because of the destruction of resident bacteria by antibiotics, leading to severe diarrhea and illness. Fecal transplants, which reintroduce a normal bacteria population into the gut, have shown tremendous promise in treating this disease, which kills thousands of persons annually.

In addition to their work involving the understanding and mapping of our resident bacterial population, researchers are working on areas such as coronary artery disease, allergies, asthma, inflammatory bowel disease, autoimmune diseases, pharmacokinetics, obesity, autism, and other poorly understood disease processes. The microbiome interacts with our bodies in many ways, most of which are not yet fully understood.

It is probable that our relationships with the vast numbers of bacteria that inhabit our body are crucial to maintaining our health. Scientists refer to the biome as another vital "organ." It is invisible, but it is all over you, and especially inside you. It does not derive from human cell lines. It is composed of trillions of microbes. The clinical significance of this "new vital organ" could change medicine.

Leaders should be aware of microbiome research because it will change many aspects of medicine. How can this be a way for the health system to reach out and understand the unique individuals, n = 1? What are the opportunities and challenges to microbiome diagnosis and treatment introduction into healthcare systems?

Deeper understanding of the genome and intracellular mechanics will change medicine. The powerful tools of computational biology and genetic sequencing are providing new insights. Recent research in the genetics of cancer has demonstrated that at the cellular and genetic level, there are similarities between cancers of different organs. These similarities create a deeper understanding of the genetic and cellular basis for cancer. There is a movement to consider classification of cancer by biochemical and genetic mechanisms rather than by organ system of origin.[21]

It is the understanding of the genetic mechanisms of disease as well as a deeper appreciation of intracellular mechanics and protein chemistry that is changing how we consider different disease states. One of the observations being made in the rigorous analysis of the genetic and cellular changes of each individual's cancer cells is that there are a multitude of changes, many of which are unique to that individual.[22] With advances in computational biology, this deep understanding of genetics and cellular mechanics will require customization of treatment at the n = 1, unique individual level.

How will health systems and physicians respond to the opportunity for customized treatment?

Many health systems are building capabilities for individualized cancer treatment based on this science of genetic individuality. It is likely that individualized treatment will be a differentiating feature for health systems.

"Quantified Self"

Larry Smarr is a mathematician and physicist involved in the development of the Internet.

More recently, he has been engaged in increasing awareness of an area of healthcare known as "quantified self." He has focused the sophisticated technology at his disposal at the University of California,—San Diego, to measure every aspect of his body's anatomy and physiology. A recent article in the *Atlantic* magazine describes Smarr's work in "quantifying Larry."[23]

Smarr makes ongoing measurements in such areas as blood, stool, genome, physiologic markers, and nutritional intake. He related the story of his bouts of abdominal pain, which were undiagnosed even after an extensive workup. Smarr used the massive computational and imaging power available to him to diagnose an inflamed sigmoid colon. Further stool, blood, and genomic testing suggested inflammatory bowel disease, not seen on his colonoscopy. Further sequential analyses of his stool bacterial population demonstrated an imbalance in certain species of bacteria coincident with his inflamed intestine. The imbalance, he postulated, was probably resulting from a past dose of antibiotics.

Smarr believes passionately that the biologic sciences are in a never-before-seen expansion of growth and understanding. As in many other fields, this understanding provides massive amounts of data; its analysis will provide profound insights into the unique individual and her health. Today, individuals and their physicians have a relatively small amount of data. According to Smarr, "Medicine has barely begun to take advantage of the million-fold increase in the amount of data available for the diagnosis and treatment of disease. Take the standard physical exam, with its weigh-in, blood pressure check, and handful of numbers gleaned from select tests performed on a blood sample. These data points give your doctor little more than a 'cartoon image' of your body. Now imagine peering at the same image drawn from a galaxy of billions of data points. The cartoon becomes a high-definition, 3-D picture, with every system and organ in the body measured and mapped in real time."

His premise is that with hundreds, millions, or perhaps even billions of data points for analysis, including not only the individual patient's measurements but those of other patients, people can make much more intelligent decisions about their healthcare choices. This understanding of the uniqueness of each individual on a biologic basis will have a profound impact on consumers' interaction with healthcare. The understanding is that, in most pharmacologic therapy, the basis for therapy has been determined on a population of heterogeneous people, while the response of a unique individual can be radically different. Consumerism will embrace this understanding of biologic uniqueness and expect healthcare to reflect its importance.

The human microbiome project, quantified self, and cancer genetic research are not "gee-whiz" snapshots of disruptive scientific innovation. They are just examples of the many areas of clinical science and basic biology that are undergoing profound changes.

Healthcare leaders must recognize that the fundamental underpinnings of human biology, and therefore of human disease, are undergoing profound and rapid change. The common thread between the disruptive biologic innovation that is occurring, whether with our "bacterial partners" or in the genetics of cancer, is our uniqueness. The $n = 1$, the unique individuality of our own biology, is the rule. Every person is unique and will expect to be treated in an individualized way.

Disruptive scientific innovation is redefining the individual and her expectations. The individual, $n = 1$, is uniquely defined by genetic makeup, microbiome, physiology, beliefs, and lifestyle within a societal context. Technological innovations allow the individual to act on her unique desires and needs.

The $n = 1$ exists within a societal context. What is the impact of these forces on how she will view healthcare? The next chapter discusses the $n = 1$ as agent of transformation of healthcare.

Chapter 4. Disruptive Scientific Innovation:

- How does the increasing speed of scientific innovation fit into the strategic plan of your organization?

- What is leadership's communication plan regarding "standardizing the practice of evidence-based medicine" and "personalized medicine?" Is this important? Why or why not?

- What are your mental models of the future for mobile computing in healthcare? What is the role of young leaders?

CHAPTER 5

The n = 1,
Unique Individual as Consumer

Joe is an active athlete with knee pain. He researches and selects the treatment modality and physician that fit his needs. His orthopedic surgeon, Dr. Jim Smith, is well prepared to meet the needs of this individual, n = 1.

Joe's Experience. "No pain, no gain," Joe always tells himself. He runs to keep in shape, but it's getting harder to manage the pain in his right knee with only over-the-counter meds. His primary care physician (PCP) has told him he has arthritis in his knee that probably started with an old sports injury. Joe feels that admitting to arthritis makes him feel older than his forty-two years, but he wants to keep active both at work and at play, and he is thinking that he will need to pursue other treatment.

Joe decides to go online to search treatment alternatives—the less invasive the better, but he is hoping for a long-term fix that gives him back his exercise routine minus the pain. He wants to find a treatment that fits his lifestyle and health status. He recently enrolled in a high-deductible health plan, so cost is an important consideration. Thankfully, he has found that shopping for treatment is now easier with the tools his insurer provides—he can compare doctors and procedures by price, quality, and patient feedback. In fact, Joe thinks, comparing doctors and treatment prices is becoming similar to comparing running shoes on Amazon.

Joe discovers online that he can purchase a DNA sequencing test to assess whether he would be a good candidate for an "arthroscopic reconstruction and genomic matched joint infusion," which sounds like the best option, but not every orthopedic surgeon performs this procedure. A link on his health insurer's web site identifies the surgeons who do, along with their pricing and patient feedback. The health insurer's network of physicians doesn't include all the orthopedic surgeons in his town, but Joe found a surgeon who seems to fit his criteria.

Joe picked Dr. Jim Smith in part because of his proximity and the importance of a short travel time. Dr. Smith's prices are competitive, and previous patients seem satisfied. Joe clicks on Dr. Smith's office site and schedules a consult for his knee assessment. Dr. Smith's office texts him back to confirm the appointment and includes an order for the lab and imaging exams to be completed beforehand.

Joe's health insurer's web site also has price comparisons for in-network lab tests and imaging centers, so he schedules them online a week before the appointment and makes arrangements to have the results added to his personal electronic health record (EHR). He found the best price for these tests was offered at an ambulatory center located in a pharmacy at a shopping center near him. The blood work was completed by a technician using a small, painless finger prick, then analyzed by a handheld device and uploaded instantaneously to servers connecting to his EHR. He added Dr. Smith to his professional access list so both he and his PCP would get his test results.

Joe shows up for his appointment with Dr. Smith and feels a connection because of the text exchange before the appointment. His old basketball injury in college involved minor surgery and rehabilitation, but that was the last time Joe needed anything other than routine primary care. Joe brings along a printout of the research he has conducted on the web about his various treatment options in case his first choice doesn't work out. He wants to be as prepared as possible for the discussion because time off from work is important. His first priority is to be ready for the annual 10K race in which he traditionally competes. It is also important to find the least expensive option, which probably will mean conducting rehabilitation at home, and to minimize his time off.

His discussion with Dr. Smith narrows his choice to two courses of treatment. Traditional arthroscopic surgery will cost $7,250, of which Joe will pay the first $5,000 and a 20 percent copay on the balance. He will have to take off two weeks from work and then undergo rehabilitation three times a week for four weeks. He will likely be able to resume running in six to eight weeks. Dr. Smith has performed more than 400 of these surgeries with highly satisfied patients and high-quality results.

Joe's second option is a new procedure that involves injecting a genetically matched infusion after arthroscopic revision. Dr. Smith has completed forty of these procedures, with promising results. The recovery time is longer, but Joe should still be able to compete in the 10K. The rehabilitation is more intense, but he likes the idea of using "video game therapy" for his home-based rehabilitation. The videos are geared to athletes and make the rehabilitation sessions competitive and fun.

The insurance company requires prior approval for this procedure, and the cost of surgery is $12,500. Joe is still responsible for the first $5,000 and has the same 20 percent copay. Joe decides that he wants to pursue this approach if he has a genetic match. He understands that his complete genome mapping will be added to his EHR.

Joe receives approval from his insurance company after Dr. Smith recommends him as a good candidate for the new procedure based on his age and health status. The surgery is performed the following week on an outpatient basis. Joe is given a web link for post-surgical care instructions and has a Skype appointment with Dr. Smith in two days to check on his progress.

After he comes home, he has his leg elevated, with ice on the incision. He has been told to look for inflammation or infection. Although he was supposed to remove the ice pack after an hour, he falls asleep, and when he wakes up the incision is sore and red. He isn't sure if infection is the cause of redness—because of the ice, the area feels cold. He calls Dr. Smith's office, and the physician assistant asks Joe to take a photo of the area with his iPhone and send it to her. After fifteen minutes, he receives a text saying that the ice could have caused a "cold burn," which will resolve itself spontaneously; if the redness is still there after an hour, he should call for an appointment.

Joe starts his home-based rehabilitation the following week. He has tiny sensors placed in appropriate locations and a connector to his smartphone, so his progress can be uploaded. He works with the physical therapist in Dr. Smith's office to find the exercises paced for his own progress and personal training objectives, and together they adjust the frequency. Joe tracks his progress online and shares it with the physical therapist.

After four weeks of home-based therapy and a follow-up visit with Dr. Smith, he is released to start light running for four weeks; following another visit to Dr. Smith, he should be ready to train for the 10K.

Months later, at the starting line for the 10K, Joe feels as if his mantra is "no pain." His training went well, and he is looking forward to improving his time. He looks over the crowd, sees Dr. Smith, and gives him a thumbs-up.

Dr. Jim Smith's Perspective. Dr. Smith checks his e-mail and sees that a runner is seeking a consult to see if a genetically matched joint infusion and arthroscopic reconstruction will work for a painful right knee. Jim is a runner himself, so he knows that Joe will want to have as much functionality as possible in the knee. The procedure has shown promising results for high-performing athletes as well as weekend warriors, as long as there is minimal damage to the area.

It will be important to check Joe's DNA and obtain an MRI. His e-mail confirms that these tests have been scheduled and he's been given access to Joe's EHR. He will review this information in the next few days to ensure no other additional tests are required. Dr. Smith sends Joe a text to let him know that he is looking forward to meeting him; he also asks about his prior sports injury and his preferred workout routine.

Joe seems to be a good candidate for the new treatment, which allows an athlete to have more mobility. He is younger than many of his patients with arthritis, and he is otherwise healthy, is not overweight, and has no chronic conditions that might influence a successful recovery.

Dr. Smith receives an e-mail when Joe's test results are in his EHR. The MRI images show that the deterioration in Joe's knee hasn't progressed so far as to prevent the infusion option, and that he has a genetic match based on the DNA tests. He asks his assistant to make the appointment for surgery on an outpatient basis as soon as he has an opening. He also copies his physical therapist to schedule a pre-op visit with Joe to explain how his rehabilitation can be done at home using video game therapy and online tracking.

The surgery seemed to go well, and Jim videotaped the procedure so Joe and his wife could watch it. His assistant gives Joe's wife the link to the web site with post-operative care instructions during the surgery so she could review the information and ask any questions she has while he is in recovery. Joe can review the instructions that are delivered by a nurse avatar when he is home and e-mail any questions on his care plan to the assistant. The video of his surgery was uploaded so Joe can watch it.

On the day after surgery, Dr. Smith's assistant tells him that Joe called about redness near the incision area. He was concerned about infection until she told him that Joe had fallen asleep with the ice on the incision and developed a "cold burn" that resolved itself.

Dr. Smith believes it is important for his patients' satisfaction and recovery that he monitor them post-surgery. He is able to track his patients efficiently with the help of technology, and he encourages updates on their progress via text, website, or videoconference.

But nothing beats seeing one of his patients back to full activity in person. On the day of the race, he seeks Joe out at the starting line and smiles as he gives him a big thumbs-up. He plans to stay behind Joe during the race just long enough to check out Joe's knee function (and his handiwork), and then he is off and running to the finish line.

The Empowered Consumer

The case of Joe and Dr. Smith is retail healthcare with an informed consumer and a retail-savvy physician. The case is not intended to predict orthopedic advances. Joe was able to balance desired results with price, convenience, and satisfaction, and he chose the best fit with his preferences. Dr. Smith used the technology to give his patient the desired care experience.

Consumers are treated as unique individuals in every other retail market; books, groceries, travel, or any other retail offerings are customized to the unique consumer. The expectations continue to grow as new products and services catering to individual needs are rapidly being developed. The imperative for those selling in the retail market is to know the individual as thoroughly as possible. The sources of information about us as consumers are mind-boggling. The analytics used to individualize our preferences are extraordinarily sophisticated.

In healthcare, technological innovation is providing individuals with tools and information to make healthcare choices. Biological innovation is deepening their understanding of the importance of their individuality. These forces create the technologically empowered and biologically unique $n = 1$.

The $n = 1$ exists in the social context of healthcare. Risk transference has created a new relationship of individuals with healthcare. This financially incented, technologically empowered, and biologically unique $n = 1$ is transforming healthcare.

How will the $n = 1$ as consumers of healthcare behave?

Individual Healthcare Beliefs and Values

Each individual has a mental model of healthcare. Each person is unique, with a corresponding value system that applies to his perception of health. The unique perceptions of healthcare frame and filter all the other elements of consumer behavior. For example, there are strong differences in perceptions in areas such as death and dying, preventive testing to determine disease, using "best practice" medicine, and the practice of "team medicine." These perceptual and value-based differences are deeply seated in each consumer.

Many of the n = 1 feel alienated from institutions. They view government, banks, and health systems with suspicion. This varies by individual and is a factor for healthcare providers. Healthcare solutions providing individual transparency and choice are likely to be most successful. This sense of alienation is but one of a multitude of individual beliefs healthcare organizations must understand.

End-of-life care is powerfully impacted by personal and family beliefs and behavior. Most healthcare leaders agree about the importance of end-of-life care decisions. Healthcare costs for an individual are the highest in the last six months of his life. Frequently the costs are for services that do not enhance or prolong life. Death and dying, end-of-life care, and advance directives are an emotionally charged area of behavior and values. No matter what the payment models are in the future, these issues must be addressed.

Healthcare is not just a purchased commodity. Consumers interacting with the healthcare delivery system have a clear and strongly held views from a values and belief basis. Transparency of information and ability to choose are beneficial in bringing treatment choices in congruence with an individual's unique value system. The ability to choose is important for the healthcare consumer. The consumer prefers healthcare that provides transparency and choice.

Many consumers value choice. They want to manage their own healthcare services so that they can choose according to their beliefs. It is a principle of the unique individual, n = 1, to have the freedom of choice: his choice may be poor, but it is his. The demise of 1990s-era managed care is testimony to the danger of concepts that constrain his healthcare choices.

Many times, an individual's beliefs will be driven by inadequate or inaccurate information. For instance, understanding the risk-benefit of diagnostic or treatment options can be difficult. Developing educated healthcare consumers will be an important challenge no matter the payment model. Educating and providing information to the n = 1 will be an opportunity for innovators.

Healthcare leadership must understand the types of unique consumers. These "market segments" can be identified in a multitude of ways. Many organizations are using predictive analytics and massive available databases to deepen their understanding of the consumer market segments.

These consumers are buying healthcare services in new ways.

Healthcare consumers are buying two broad categories of services: preventive services to bring them wellness and healthcare services to treat illness.

The Consumer Buys Prevention

Consumers buy prevention services to get health and wellness. This is a prime example of an individual's belief systems regarding healthcare. The values and belief systems that influence how a consumer views his own wellness influences his consumption of healthcare services. The CDC estimates that 60 percent of healthcare costs are engendered by personal behavior decisions.[24] Understanding this aspect of behavior is important.

There is an assumption that risk transference to individuals will provide incentives for their healthy behavior. No matter what the incentives might be, deeply held beliefs influence how each patient manages his health. His deeply held belief systems can support behavior that damages his health; he may disregard scientific evidence and the advice of trusted professionals. Therefore, as the transformation of healthcare occurs, it must be with the knowledge that the n = 1 has a fundamental requirement that healthcare must be in congruence with his values and beliefs. The understanding of these values and beliefs is crucial to the engagement of individuals with their own healthcare costs and quality. Addressing these belief and behavioral issues is key to managing healthcare costs.

Wellness programs are an important focus for entrepreneurs in healthcare. Selling apps or services to consumers is more straightforward than selling to provider organizations. The advent of high-deductible health plans creates a potential incentive for the individual. Wellness programs have produced mixed value over the years. The ability to prevent illness and save money has been historically difficult to document in most programs. Recently, companies have provided wellness programs to employees in conjunction with these plans to help control their own expenses. Most offer some financial incentives for participation in such activities as exercise, smoking cessation, or weight loss.

Many new companies have created useful apps to provide prevention guidance to consumers. Apps can involve diet, weight, exercise, sleep, and meditation to encourage healthful living. The apps primarily provide information, measurement, and guidance, and not specific recommendations or treatment plans.

Wellness and prevention services are important in population health. In a situation where a provider organization is responsible for the healthcare costs of an entire population over time, it is prudent to keep that population healthy.

Addressing the personal behavior decisions in nutrition, substance abuse, and exercise will have a significant impact on healthcare costs. The belief systems that promote a healthy lifestyle, or not, may determine the long-term success of healthcare cost control and the economic success of those holding the risk. Innovation in the area of individual engagement in lifestyle change will be as crucial as in any other area of healthcare.

The Consumer Buys Healthcare

Consumers will have more "skin in the game" with healthcare purchases in the future. The transference of risk for healthcare services from the government and employers to individuals is happening quickly. The economic responsibility of the consumer will have a profound impact on the healthcare system.

Consumers armed with information regarding their medical conditions, provider quality, and price will be making purchasing decisions. Their choices will be made within narrow provider networks. The decision-making of consumers will be enhanced by input from other consumers with similar medical issues who have visited providers in the network.

As in online retailing, evaluation of physician and provider services by other consumers is increasingly available. Services are available that "crawl" through the online worlds of Twitter, Facebook, and other social networking sites to find "mentions" of healthcare organizations or physicians. The "mentions" are then graphically displayed so the frequency of the same comment is represented, as well as the number of views.

Transparency of patient satisfaction, presented like online product reviews, will create angst and controversy. In fact, there have been lawsuits by physicians against patients who posted negative online reviews. It is unclear how consumer information tools from other industries will work in healthcare. It is likely that all these tools will be tried. They will be adopted by certain segments of consumers and providers, and they will continue to evolve. What is certain is that they won't go away.

Consumer choices will further be enhanced by the accumulation of additional cost-quality information in the network. Much larger databases will further allow comparison of treatment options as well as cost and quality. This retail medicine will focus on consumers. They will choose their healthcare options, and they will organize the health system around their choices.

There are theoretical limits to the effectiveness of this approach. Once the deductible is met, the consumer can be relatively insensitive to the price. People with chronic illness who must organize their own healthcare may not be capable of shopping effectively. The ability of individuals who may have limited ability to make wise purchasing decisions may also be a limit on retail medicine.

The fundamental strategy of informing consumers and placing them at risk will continue to grow. Its impact is likely to reduce utilization. This reduction may be of both appropriate and inappropriate utilization. It is the individual's choice.

The transference of risks to consumers is a boon to innovators. There are opportunities to substitute lower-cost care processes, provide more information to consumers, assess provider performance, and many other services. Disruptive new entrants will seek these opportunities.

Many consumers will engage with health systems that provide population health services. These provide a continuum of care for patients within the context of a closed or closely coordinated network. This allows patients to access care in a closely coordinated fashion.

In population healthcare systems, the risk is transferred to the provider, who is paid a set fee to care for a patient or a population a people for a fixed unit of time. This can range from a large group of people over a year to a single procedure for one patient. A single payment that is fixed provides the transference of risk. The incentive is to provide the most effective care at the best cost. If the cost is less than the payment, the provider benefits; if it's more, the provider loses.

The n = 1 will receive coordinated-care experience in a health system that will be reaching out to provide services for both wellness and prevention with the goal of maintaining the individual's health so he will not require medical services. This can be particularly advantageous to those with chronic illness, the elderly, and those who have difficulty in purchasing in a retail market.

Organizations that are currently involved in population health have demonstrated the importance of understanding the individuality of each consumer within their population. Health systems will be providing information to individuals to assist them in managing their own health. Prevention and wellness services will be important. Connection of consumers to their online personal health information is an important part of care management.

Population health will also create opportunities for innovators. They will provide health systems with assessments of the disease burden of populations, patient education programs, and care process coordination, among other services. Health systems will drive much of the innovation, as they are at risk.

Retail and population health are artificial distinctions for the consumer markets. They will blend together. Risk transference to both individuals and providers will be increased. Those holding the insurance risk—government and employers—will be continuing to shift risk to contain costs.

This all comes together with n = 1: unique individuals as consumers as the transformative force of healthcare.

This has several important implications:

- Financial incentives for individuals to be effective consumers of healthcare are increasing.
- Financial incentives for providers to take risk for groups of individuals is increasing.
- Information in easily usable forms for consumers is rapidly increasing.
- Unique individuals have their own set of values and beliefs regarding healthcare, which they will continue to reflect in their behaviors.
- Consumers have increasingly sophisticated tools to evaluate and choose healthcare services.
- The revolutionary advances occurring in biological sciences underscore the uniqueness of the individual and the complexity of each person.
- The n = 1 consumerism is a potent trend, further enabled and accelerated by trends in digitization and disruptive scientific innovation.

The next section of the book is about the provider's opportunities given these forces.

Chapter 5. Consumer:

- What are three ways retail medicine will impact your organization in the next three years?

- Do social network referral models like Airbnb and Lyft have applicability to healthcare? If so, how?

- Do your targeted consumers expect your organization's focus to be on illness care? Wellness care? Both?

- How should the brand promise of your organization be influenced by the answer to the above question?

- How does the strategic plan and budget of your healthcare organization explicitly reflect the answer to the question about the balance between illness care and wellness care?

PART III

Meeting the Needs
of n = 1

The transformative forces in healthcare enable the n = 1 to demand different features and benefits from every healthcare organization. New competencies and imperatives are required for organizational success. Existing organizations must develop new competencies and eliminate old practices. New entrants, competing with legacy healthcare organizations, will be building from scratch, meeting n = 1 expectations in new ways. Leaders must develop a clear framework for the necessary competencies to be developed in their people and in their organization.

Leaders must create the organizational capacity and processes for new competencies. The focus is always on the needs of the n = 1.

CHAPTER 6

Imperatives and Competencies

The same forces that have transformed other industries are leading inexorably to a restructuring of healthcare's incentives affecting consumers, providers, insurers, and employers. Key imperatives identified from industries that have faced similar forces will serve as a framework for the transformed organization. This is a "jumping-off point" for questions regarding strategies and business plans that will transform the organization.

Each organization will develop its own set of imperatives. Our research shows that most important are to:

- Articulate a clear mission, vision, and values based on the organization's heritage.
- Develop and maintain a learning organization mindset and infrastructure.
- Institutionalize translation of innovation.
- Understand the business model of the organization.
- Operate innovative people and leadership development strategies.
- Communicate effectively.
- Monitor and interact with the external environment, especially customers.
- Consider data as the foundation for transformation.
- Collaborate effectively.

The successful transformation of organizations requires a number of specific competencies. Our research demonstrates that there is one competency that is decidedly the most important: CEO leadership.

Leadership by the CEO, or by the CEO and a strong board, is essential. We could find no evidence of successful transformation of an organization, in any industry, without it. The transformation of organizations is difficult even with strong CEO leadership; it is impossible without that leadership.

"Are you up for this?"

This is the question that each CEO should look in the mirror and ask. It is extremely difficult to disrupt one's own business or industry. Many CEOs have personal or professional circumstances that preclude their complete commitment to organizational transformation. The intent of the question is not to pass judgment but to encourage self-awareness and honesty. If the CEO is not up for the transformative changes, then it will likely end poorly for all involved.

"Are you up for this?"

Are you seeing the changes of healthcare clearly and accurately? What will it mean for you?

Are you deepening your understanding of change through conversations with others, who may view it through a different lens? There is no place for wishful thinking. Seek out people who will challenge you.

Are you personally involved in the transformational work? Is it part of your organizational identity?

Courage is a common theme emerging from conversations with CEOs who have led organizations through difficult transformation.

"You have the courage to see things as they really are. You must let go of what you have created in the past."

Questions are often very difficult for CEOs to ask. They are expected to know the answers, and some people equate asking questions with weakness. Questions imply a CEO is not in control. CEOs do not want to appear weak or not in control, and, as a result, they will often reflect outward certainty and confidence despite their internal uncertainty. Sometimes they are in denial about their uncertainty; this is absolutely understandable—but it is dangerous.

However, it is only through questions and dialogue that a CEO can create a map of transition for transformation of their organization. This takes courage.

No CEO does this alone. She needs to ask herself:

- Do I have the right team?
- Will the board and senior leadership assist me?
- Do they share my passion and vision?
- Have I asked each of them, "Are you up for this?" Do I believe their answers?

What is your mechanism to help members of your team with their professional insecurity? Each CEO will have her own way to work with her leadership team to manage this insecurity.

Looking in the mirror and asking, "Are you up for this?" is an act of self-awareness. Self-awareness and intellectual integrity are requirements for a CEO in the process of transforming her organization.

The board must demonstrate their leadership for the organization, and must also ask the CEO, "Are you up for this?" In transformational times, the CEO's answer to this question is the ultimate accountability of governance.

The CEO who answers, "Yes, I am up for this!" must develop a set of organizational competencies. Many of these already exist in varying degrees within the organization. They must now fit together, like pieces of a complex puzzle, in an organizational model of transformation, molding the organization to the leader's strategic intent.

These competencies are the most frequently mentioned in conversations with transformational healthcare leaders. They are also directly comparable to the competencies developed in other transforming industries. They can be segmented in many ways, and each deserves attention.

Articulate a Clear Mission, Vision, and Values
Based on the Organization's Heritage

Leaders in the midst of transformational change will consider how they provide stability and consistency for employees in the organization. Many will not have an understanding of the rationale for organizational change, and they might be concerned or fearful. Frequent and consistent communication is important; however, grounding in the mission, vision, and values is critical. Very often, the mission of the organization and its values do not change.

How the organization fulfills its mission, in the context of its values and heritage, is the focus of change. If, in spite of significant transformational change, the organization's evolution seems consistent with the mission, vision, values, and heritage, the cultural acceptance of change will be stronger.

Adoption is more likely if the transformational message is a reiteration of "who we are and why we do what we do." It's well known that the most important motivator for employees is the inspiration that comes from being part of something larger than themselves. This can be a more powerful motivator than a paycheck. Because of the nature of the work and commitment, this is especially true in healthcare. Leadership, by providing a clear grounding in the mission, vision, and values, provides a "true north" for the organization. This consistency provides a level of trust required for transformational change.

The vision embraces transformational trends and how the organization aspires to meet those trends in the future. It is necessary for the vision to be broad enough to answer questions about how the organization will meet the needs of the unique individual, n = 1; population health; digitization; and disruptive innovation. Many organizations engage diverse constituencies in the development of their vision.

Communication and socialization of the mission, vision, and values are a major responsibility of senior leadership. Integrity of leadership, both in talk and in action, provide the trust for change.

The urgency of transformation or the frenetic nature of the market-place should not interfere with the creation of the infrastructure of trust created by leaders living the mission, vision, and values.

Develop and Maintain a Learning Organization Mindset and Infrastructure

Health systems with a rapid-cycle process for adopting innovation throughout the organization will have the most success. This is easily seen in the experience of organizations in nonhealth industries facing highly competitive, knowledge-intense markets. Organizations like Apple and Google use the intellectual capital of their people as a strategic asset, and they identify and reduce barriers to innovation. General Electric historically has institutionalized with management systems the identification and spread of innovation across industries and businesses.

Innovation is not about discovering the next "big new thing." It is most often about how existing processes and technology are com-bined in novel ways to produce value. This recombination is often best done by those "closest to the action." Thus, bringing together the people involved in healthcare to recombine pieces of healthcare processes is what creates value.

The term "expert-to-expert learning" has been used to describe learning organizations, which become adept at identifying opportuni-ties and bringing together experts to identify innovative solutions. The organizations provide a nurturing environment that encourages this process. Naturally, people appreciate being called experts, espe-cially when they are treated as such. These experts feed off the expert-ise and experience of their colleagues. Expert-to-expert learning is particularly important in healthcare because of the predominately provincial nature of healthcare practice. The respectful relationships of experts can break down the provincial walls.

As innovations are developed and tested, the preparation for adoption should be made. Adoption of innovation across scale will produce maximal value. The rationale for vertical and horizontal integration is to achieve scale, a major advantage of which is to reap the benefits of innovation in one part of the organization and spread it across the entirety. This won't simply happen. It must be designed into the organization and modeled by the senior leaders. The design must include a culture of spread, plus management systems supporting innovation.

In general, healthcare has a long history of "not invented here." Over the last decade or so, we have seen growing interest in evidence-based medicine, but even with this interest and a sincere desire to do the right thing, the spread of innovation can be slow.

One health system with which we are familiar had developed an innovative approach to blood conservation during cardiovascular surgery. Surgeons had conducted extensive research and published peer-reviewed articles about their ability to reduce morbidity and mortality by managing and reducing transfusions. Now these procedures are well accepted in the field. However, in the beginning, even though they worked in a hospital that was part of a health system with a dozen other heart programs, the innovation took nearly seven years to be adopted throughout the health system. Health systems, medical groups, and other provider organizations will not be successful in the future if a process innovation like this takes seven years for adoption across a system.

Another important aspect of creating a learning organization is attracting talent and appropriately using the intellectual capacities of its people. Particularly in healthcare, the appreciation and rewarding of expertise is a powerful incentive to become part of an organization. As health systems and medical groups become larger, there are substantial possibilities for talented experts to grow professionally in the organization.

The innovation of the future will not only be scientific discovery; much like the transfusion story above, it will be about innovation of processes led by those experts closest to the action.

Talent in the future will come from many non-traditional sources. Technology experts and data scientists are attracted to organizations that value innovation and expert-to-expert learning. A commitment to a learning organization model will be an asset for attracting the right people.

Institutionalize the Translation of Innovation

Providers on the front line may find it difficult to engage in the implementation of innovation, even if it can lead to improvements in productivity for the broader organization. They may not view productivity as a problem, since they might view their unit or domain as working quite well. Therefore, "selling them" on an organization-wide productivity solution may be difficult. The challenges of implementing electronic medical records (EMRs) is still a fresh memory in many organizations, which might make additional large-scale innovation difficult in the near future. What can be learned from the spread of EMRs that will help in the future? EMRs are just the beginning of innovation and transformation. The organization and its people must become proficient at change.

In health systems, organic internal innovation occurs continuously. The transformative forces and social context are providing impetus for innovators and entrepreneurs external to healthcare organizations. They often do not understand the complex dynamics within the health system, and may not have a clear idea of the actual problem. Many technology innovators come from the retail world and are very customer-(patient)-centric. At one recent technology conference, a frustrated healthcare technology entrepreneur described the health system provider culture as a "calcified hairball," meaning that the provider culture was difficult to penetrate: it had a culture of entitlement and was slow to implement change. In the opinion of many external and even internal innovators, healthcare has significant challenges translating innovation into practice.

"An open letter to health entrepreneurs" in *Rock Health*[25] from a young emergency physician provides insight into how some physicians think about those healthcare technology entrepreneurs. He writes:

"There are two fundamental differences between how you and I think. First, my threshold for allowing error is insanely high. My job doesn't give me the luxury of beta testing or iterating. When your work is faulty, your site might go down, customers might get angry, you might lose money. When my work is faulty, people die. If you want me to use something new, it needs to have an error ratio at least equal to, if not significantly better than, the status quo, preferably with data to back up that assertion.

"Second, if you're going about the product development by thinking, 'This would be cool,' instead of 'This fulfills a pressing clinical need better than anything else out there,' you're doing it wrong.

"I hope this helps clarify why I view just about every new healthcare startup with a cautious eye. I'm not against change at all; in fact, if you come barging into my domain without adequately considering patient safety and product quality, I will lose all respect for you. I get it; we both belong to peculiar and somewhat arrogant fields, and we both want what's best according to our worldviews. But let's try to meet eye to eye or else we will get nowhere."

Aaron Martin recently came to healthcare from Amazon, where he worked on the development of self-publishing and the Kindle. He brings to healthcare the excitement of technological innovation. When asked about his impressions of the differences between a large health system and Amazon, he focuses on similarities and opportunities:

- Healthcare is about the use of the scientific method: creation of a hypothesis based on observations and controlled experiments in which data is collected, which results in the development of a treatment;
- Standardization of clinical practice is bringing increased discipline to the experimentation;

- The focus on the healthcare customer's total experience, a passion of Amazon, is often not a priority in healthcare. This will change, as the n = 1 is more discriminating;
- Engaging in small experiments with measurement of value based on a core hypothesis of value creation will accelerate change. The cycle is Build-Measure-Learn;
- Be alert to where value is added and what triggers a customer to adopt a solution: it might surprise you.

Aaron describes how the value to clients of the car-sharing service Uber is beyond price and convenience. The app does more than summon a car; it shows the car on your mobile device as it approaches you. You see your car coming, and you know that the car is on its way and the driver's name, thereby alleviating the anxiety that typically exists when a client calls a cab company, places an order, and *hopes* a cab is coming, never knowing its status until arrival. Uber has identified customer pain: "Where's my car?" An unexpected value of Uber is relief of this anxiety, which creates "stickiness" with the client for the service. Uber "discovered" this customer pain by the "small batch innovation" process described above.[26] Aaron and other entrepreneurs are working to bring to healthcare the same small-batch/lean-product development approach used to develop new products and services by technology firms.

Many tech entrepreneurs use a business reference, *The Lean Startup*,[27] which has broader application to rapid-cycle innovation in any setting. The thesis is that entrepreneurship is management. Traditional management systems were developed to build "things." The Lean Startup management approach is geared to uncertainty and what is termed "validated learning." The entrepreneurs run frequent small experiments that allow them to test each element of their vision. Innovation accounting measures progress, sets milestones, and prioritizes work.

It is clear that healthcare will be identifying new management systems to engage in rapid innovation with entrepreneurs embedded in the organization. As health systems bring in talent from other industries, the processes to manage transformation will evolve.

Most large health systems either have or are considering the development of an innovation institute, innovation accelerator, or innovation venture fund. The purpose of an innovation accelerator can vary from adoption to diversification of revenue. Many organizations with a strong research mission and faculty have innovation institutes to promote internal innovation and the commercialization of it. Often these organizations will partner with other health systems, venture capital, other innovation accelerators, non-healthcare companies, and health insurers. The common theme is the commercialization of intellectual property from the research of the cutting-edge health system.

In addition, organizations invest in early- to mid-stage companies and offer the opportunity for piloting within the health system. For example, the Cleveland Clinic, Intermountain Healthcare, Tenet, Ascension, Unity Point Health, and Memorial Care Health System all participate in innovation funds. They work with early- to mid-stage companies focused on medical devices, healthcare information technology, or healthcare services. The clinical access provided is often more valuable than the monetary investment. Organizations may hold contests to identify technological solutions to specific clinical problems. They invite entrepreneurs to enter and potentially win money, investment opportunities, or clinical access.

The vision of the UCLA Institute for Innovation in Health says it will, in part, "foster, convene, and lead innovation to transform the delivery of healthcare within UCLA health and in regional, national, and global partnerships. Our goal is to radically transform the value of healthcare by building an enduring platform to accelerate innovation at UCLA that improves quality, engages patients, and reduces the net cost of care."

There are as many different innovation institutes, accelerators, incubators, and translators as there are organizations, and all are trying to achieve similar outcomes. The focus of some is more on commercializing internal innovations, while others are identifying investment and partnering opportunities with external innovators.

The ability to be close to the introduction of innovative new approaches has potential for new revenue streams and first-to-market advantages. The ability to have a learning organization that can translate innovations from all sources into changes in process and improvement in clinical care is even more important. The capabilities of a learning organization and a translator of innovation go hand in hand.

Understand the Business Model of the Organization

This is likely one of the areas of most difficult transformation. For decades, the mechanism of reimbursement has been fee-for-service, with various adjustments for certain types of services. Retail medicine and population-based medicine in all their various forms are bringing different incentives and payment models. Most healthcare organizations receive a multitude of different payment schemes that complicate business-model understanding.

In a planning exercise, the top 2 percent of leaders in a large organization were asked, "How do we make money in the organization?" Their answers required a modest level of specificity, such as the payer, service, location, and patient type. The leaders were then asked to write the answers without consulting their colleagues. The responses were compared with the CFO's answer. The relative lack of understanding and agreement of how the business model works was revealing, and it became a good starter discussion of the long-range financial plan and scenarios for the future. Graphic representations of the areas of profitability over time can be a powerful discussion tool. This can be a useful exercise for the board of directors, but only if the CEO has done the appropriate preparation and is ready for the follow-up questions. The point is not to embarrass anyone, but to highlight the difficulty in complex organizations to pinpoint exactly where the most significant transactions of money for value occur.

Cardiology practices serve as an example of rapid revenue change. In 2009, CMS reduced reimbursement for nuclear medicine by 22 percent, echocardiography by 13 percent, and cardiovascular stress tests by 6.2 percent (based on CPT codes 78452, 93306, and 93015). In a very short time, practices that had depended on nuclear medicine studies needed to find new strategies to generate practice margins, which precipitated a movement of cardiology practices to hospital employment. These types of changes are being repeated over and over again.

These "how *exactly* do we make money" questions, are important to incorporate in discussions of transformational imperatives, since health systems and physicians participate in a multitude of payment schemes, each having differential incentives and margins. As the old saying goes, "If you don't know where you are, it's hard to know where you're going." The future will be much less forgiving to those who do not know exactly how they are generating their revenue and their margins. Not only will the revenues likely be less, but also the purchasers will be more discriminating about value. For example, the implications of the retail business model will be profound. The requirement for transparency of competitive pricing will be a challenge for large and complex health systems.

The growth of high-deductible plans and retail services influences the consumer's purchasing behavior. The magnitude of cash collections of health systems and physicians will change. It is estimated by Accenture that patient collections for retail services will grow nationally by 7 percent to $3.7 billion in 2018.[28] The current processes in most organizations for revenue cycle and cash collections were not created to manage this number of retail patient payments. There will be a strong impetus to gather information about insurance coverage and obtain payment at the time of service.

The business-model implications of a population-health model of payment are also potentially significant. In the vertically integrated model of population health in its purest form, there is a single payment for a population over time. Allocation of the medical expenses is the "internal economy," requiring allocation of payments to the hospital, physician, drugs, outpatient, and other services required to care for the population. Models include an ownership model, with internally agreed upon "transfer price," for services with the owned parts of a system; another is a contractual network with formal negotiated service contracts. There is every model between these two.

There are advantages and disadvantages to the degree of owner-ship integration in healthcare population management. High levels of integration, as at Kaiser, allow for standardization of process, expense control, and brand differentiation. On the other hand, this model is expensive to replicate, is difficult to manage if there is a downturn in business, and can become bureaucratic. Networked models can be difficult to differentiate, standardize, and manage. There is no right answer other than great leadership and management of whatever model works in the market.

Most organizations will have a mixed, highly integrated and net-worked model that will be flexible to manage and expand. Flexibility is important, as there is uncertainty in the speed and development of the population health market. The overall success of the integrated model is contingent on the success of managing the overall per capita payment and the ability to manage the internal transfer payments to the components, such as physicians and hospitals, so that their strate-gic goals can be realized. The negotiations between the Permanente Medical group and the Kaiser Health Plan reflect that healthy dynamic tension. Provider-owned health plans have difficult "internal market" discussions reconciling the price of premium marketability and growth with the expectations for payment to the owner facilities and physicians. There is no shortcut or easy way to manage this inter-nal market.

One of the business model challenges for traditional fee-for-service providers organizing to take population health risk by verti-cally integrating is to remove waste. For example, as the bed days per thousand decline and there are fewer procedures, how does the overall system meet the expectations of the component participants? One person's waste is another person's profit.

Growth is fundamental to the business model in transitioning from fee-for-service to population health. Increasing the number of people served and "touched" by the system can potentially mitigate the decline in the profitability per person. It also allows the spread of risk over a larger number of people, which is important from an actu-arial standpoint. Leaders must develop clear plans to accomplish this goal. After all, every other organization in your market is thinking the same thing. How will your organization differentiate itself in the areas that matter to the n = 1 consumers?

A large, integrated medical group practice that owned a hospital and a health plan was purchased by a large investor-owned insurance company, which planned to offer a staff-model HMO option in the market. They did not own any other provider organizations. Early in the relationship, the leadership of the medical group identified a key need for improvements in imaging, particularly with access to their emergency room. New CT and MRI devices had been built into the capital expense budget of the hospital.

Upon seeing the request for a multimillion-dollar capital expense, the leadership of the insurance company wanted to know why there was a need for such capital expenditures: "Why can't you just buy imaging services from another provider?" The medical group explained that, when people came to the emergency room, they needed immediate care—not to be sent across town to another provider.

The capital expense did not fit into the budget formula of the insurance company. The health insurance business does not require many fixed-asset capital investments. Several years later, the insurance company, the medical group, and the hospital completely "disintegrated." The complexity of mixed business models and differing cultures was causing effort and energy beyond the value created by vertical integration. The evolving payment schemes cause changes not only in business models, but also in the culture of the organization.

Three-year financial plans expose questions and assumptions about fundamental issues such as program profitability, resource allocation, and capital planning. The next thirty-six months are impossible to predict with precision; however, by discussing the scenarios, the management team (and board of directors) will be able to have an array of models and options to deploy as things do play out.

Health systems with long-standing ownership of their own health plan have extensive experience in combining the business models of health insurance and healthcare-delivery systems. Scenario planning will assist the management team in understanding the implications and assumptions of the differing business models.

Operate Effective People Strategies and Leadership Development

The newly appointed CEO of a health system was given the gift of a coach by the board. The coach was Ram Charan. The CEO met with Charan to develop a coaching relationship. Five minutes into the first meeting, Charan instructed, "Take out a piece of paper and write *people*." He paused. "Then write *people*." He again paused. "Then write *people*." Charan leaned forward and said, "Look closely at your paper. If you get those three things right, you will do fine as a CEO."

It makes no difference if you are leading a health system, medical group, or insurance company; it all boils down to the people. An organization is an aggregate of the intellectual capital and energy of the its people.

Two or three decades ago, the organizational structure and management systems of health systems, medical groups, and insurance companies were relatively straightforward. Today the complexity of the market and the evolution of organizations require much more complex talent planning.

As your organization charts the future, how are you identifying new skills and competencies that are required for success? The new skills include data scientists, community outreach professionals, preventive health experts, social networking technologists, communications, and data security professionals. Many future competencies may not even exist today.

A local hospital leadership team, part of a larger health system, was planning a new hospital in their community. Great attention was given to facility design, aesthetics, and functional planning. The leadership of the health system came for a project review. Their tough questions were about the adequacy of the staffing and physician leadership plans, not about the facility construction. This caught the local leaders flatfooted. The health system leaders were much more interested in the people plans than the building plan. They knew it was the people who would make the new facility successful.

A health system recruited a senior executive who had been closely involved in the development and marketing of the Kindle at Amazon. The health system CEO wanted a new perspective on customers, the n = 1. The system leadership turned the transformational process for engaging customers over to his different mind-set. The new senior executive and his "out of healthcare" software development team took on the problem with a different perspective and a different set of tools in their toolbox. Talented executives with different perspectives spot the opportunities to serve the n = 1 in different ways.

The roles in health systems can change rapidly. Recent conversations with Chief Medical Information Officers (CMIO) indicate their jobs are changing as installations of EHRs are completed. How the role of the CMIOs is evolving is not clear. CMIOs feel as if the health systems are saying, "Now that the EHR is installed, just let it run, and thanks for your help." How are health systems reimagining their organization as it evolves? How are they retraining and repositioning existing talent? How are the leaders communicating the talent needs of the organization?

How are health systems explicitly attracting new talent? Some skills, like those of data scientists, are difficult to find in any industry. Perhaps they may be grown from within or recruited from out of industry. Detailed plans for talent management should include not only the types of competencies required, but also the types of compensation, incentives, and work environment these skilled professionals may require.

Being clear about talent needs will assist in recruiting. Discussions with successful non-healthcare technological innovators and entrepreneurs suggest that many have an altruistic desire to "do good." Many of them feel healthcare creates an excellent environment for this type of talent.

As we have discussed, leadership development is critical for transforming organizations. Leadership styles that were successful in the past may not be successful in the future transformed health system. Organizational demands, complexities, and diversity of roles will require different types of leadership.

Health systems, which traditionally have been headed by hospital leaders, will require more diversity of experiential background. As the demographics of the workforce change, significant changes in leadership style will be required. Many forward-looking health systems have made significant investments in leadership development. The leaders in these health systems know the world is changing, and they want to bring those skills to the transformed system. What are the skills needed to be successful with the n = 1 as a consumer, purchaser, or patient?

Physician-leadership development is critical. Health systems and medical groups will depend on strong physician leadership to meet the challenges of clinical transformation and payment changes. This is an area of critical need in every health system and medical group. Physicians will lead the restructuring of clinical processes to serve the needs and desires of the n = 1. Physicians will lead their colleagues in transformation. Most physicians are fully engaged in their practice and aren't considering the changes required of them. These physicians can be angry, disengaged, or frustrated. Physician leaders must develop the skills to transition these colleagues. Strong and skilled physician leadership is an important differentiating feature of successful organizations. Every healthcare organization should be asking how much resources they should place into physician leadership development.

In addition to the identification and recruitment of new talent, there is a need to effectively manage the existing people. Talent management is evolving. Many health systems and medical groups have significant cultural inertia against performance-management strategies because of the culture based in professionalism of physicians, nurses, and other clinical professionals. The notion of corporate-style talent and performance management is alien.

Effective performance-based management systems assess, document, and provide feedback to individuals. Healthcare, for the most part, has not had a culture of disciplined assessment of individual performance. Professional culture and collegiality inhibit the ability to rigorously assess performance and provide feedback. Individual performance-based management systems can be problematic in a team-oriented, collegial, and professional culture. The people system will function as it is designed to function, so the talent management and senior leadership team must design thoughtfully for the future. What are the performance objectives for serving unique individuals or a population health client? What performance-management systems will create effective integration of institutions or physicians?

In *Leadership Pipeline*, Ram Charan discusses the ongoing need to rigorously evaluate competencies and abilities of individuals. This is not only to assure the organization's success, but also to best use their gifts. He describes a case study in which a large global organization is making a product shift, with the new product entry being planned over the next twelve months into the new country's market. The organization's executive market leader in that country has been managing an existing product line and has shown skill in managing the day-to-day operational issues arising out of an established product and business.

The leaders discussed the entry of a new product and the people requirements. The new product entry required areas like marketing, governmental approval, graphics, cultural sensitivity, new relationships, new distribution channels, and public relations. They asked key questions regarding the capability of the current leader to execute the new product entry. After reviewing past performance evaluations in discussion with supervisors, they informed the leader that they would be moving him to another role that played to his strengths. A leader with the required competencies developed in another part of the organization was selected for the new product entry.

Leaders of healthcare organizations have come a long way in their recognition of talent and performance management. The transformation of healthcare will reconfigure many roles and responsibilities. How will talent be retrained, redeployed, and reinvigorated?

Even with talent development, significant reductions in force will likely occur in healthcare. Many roles will be changed. Look no further than publishing, music, or newspapers to see how the n = 1 has changed the roles of professionals in their organizations. How can forward-looking talent management and development programs assist in preserving the best talent in a transforming organization?

Expert Communications

In transformational times, it is impossible to over-communicate. Words matter. Communication should have a common framework, language, and words. Transformational communication is similar to a political campaign. Ideas need to be presented in ways people can understand. They must speak to the head and heart. Inspirational stories, images, and feelings are key.

Communications by leaders should never be taken for granted. The impact of words, appearances, and even expressions can be profound. Change must be communicated in a very thoughtful way. Disseminating information too rapidly can have negative consequences; trust lost because of haste or poorly conceived communication is difficult to recover, if it is recovered at all.

Frank Luntz, in his best-selling book, *Words That Work: It's Not What You Say, It's What People Hear*,[29] explains the role of language and communications in the political world. Luntz shapes the language around issues. For example, the language around "estate tax" became the "death tax," which turned a relatively arcane issue into a national hot button. "Drilling for oil" became "energy exploration." In times of transformation, healthcare leaders need to understand how their constituencies inside the organization hear their words and, as never before, how the external world of customers hears their words. This isn't "spin"; this is effective communication. Some healthcare CEOs refer to themselves as Chief Education Officer.

Leaders must find their voices regarding the key transformative forces. They must be clear about the role of the unique individual, the n = 1, and how that fits into the overall message. How is digitization changing our organization? Is the sacred trust with patients still important? Clinicians are very familiar with the concept of the individual patient. Marketing studies demonstrate that patients want to be viewed as individuals. How does this fit into our organization? What does the transformation of healthcare mean to me?

As healthcare organizations transform into large, integrated health systems, they develop a branded healthcare experience. This requires clarity about their role in serving the unique individual, n = 1. The description of this "brand promise" is delivered to both internal and external audiences. How do we serve our patients? For instance, the Providence Health and Services brand promise is in the voice of the n = 1: "Know me, care for me, and ease my way."

Internal communication of other transformative trends, such as digitization, are also important. The implementation of electronic medical records in most organizations has been challenging, with significant dissatisfaction among the clinical staff. Communication about the future use of data and how it will advance patient care is crucially important. Physicians must feel that they are providing not only a new administrative function but a path to better care. Thus, communications must continually link to the long-term goals of the organization to assist in getting through the short-term hurdles of transformation.

Monitor and Respond to the External Environment and Customers

Leaders of all organizations must have a high level of intellectual curiosity about the environment and how changes will affect their organizations. A key lesson from other industries is the importance of global market awareness. The transformative forces impacting healthcare are not unique to either the United States or healthcare. They have been impacting industry sectors, in varying degrees and speeds, for decades. The world is interconnected.

Monitoring the external environment begins with ongoing exercises of understanding societal change, facilitated by discussions with leaders from other industries. Many industry leaders have arranged for periodic meetings of their senior leadership team with their counterparts in other industries. The discussions range from how transformative forces have affected their organizations to how they view healthcare and the effect of transformative forces. Exposure of younger leaders within the organization to these exchanges can yield significant results in leadership development. The insights are eye-opening.

Innovations

The innovations occurring in digitization and disruptive scientific innovations are increasingly rapid and inexorable. The multiplier is the impact of recombination, the use of innovations from different disciplines in novel ways to solve problems in other areas. Recombination is evident in the example of Theranos, which will be explored in Chapter 10. Technology that was initially used for military field-testing for toxic biologic agents was expanded to pharmaceutical trials. Progress in nanotechnology, microfluidics, mobile communications, chemistry, genomics, predictive analytics, computer science, and other areas have come together to improve the individual patient experience in laboratory testing in healthcare.

Many of the independent technologies were not known a decade ago, let alone their aggregation into a valuable combination. Theranos will be discussed later as a disruptive new entrant to healthcare. The recombination of these separate innovations into a highly innovative new lab service will disrupt the industry. How are leaders tracking and anticipating the impact of the recombinant technologies?

A biological revolution is being driven by new insights into fundamental disease processes and treatment. Leaders must pay close attention to this revolution and determine how it may be used within a healthcare organization. This biologic revolution will change many of their clinical offerings.

Leaders must be purposefully and aggressively learning from outside innovators. How else will health system and medical group leaders stay on top of innovations in biology, predictive analytics, mobile health, healthcare apps, and disruptive innovation? How, explicitly, does the organization evaluate innovation developed elsewhere? Is there a formalized channel for innovators from outside the health system to routinely engage with the leaders?

For instance, when a senior leader explores the potential of the human microbiome, he should be asking a series of questions: Who in our organization is tracking this? What is the potential impact on our current services? How can the microbiome offer a better level of service to our individual patients? Is this something we should be tracking on a regular basis? If so, how should we track it? Who is accountable?

Advocacy

Advocacy is critically important to healthcare. The relationship between healthcare and the various levels of government continues to evolve. Outside of healthcare, other highly regulated industries such as banking and public utilities have learned how to interact with the regulatory and legislative branches of local, state, and federal governments.

Monitoring and providing input to federal and state governments is necessary as their involvement in healthcare, already large, continues to grow. Legislation such as the Affordable Care Act and the aging of the population will ensure the primacy of the government as the largest payer and rule-maker.

There are many issues about which healthcare organizations need to inform and educate policy decision-makers. We have selected three fundamental issues to highlight:

- *Regulatory barriers to the delivery of integrated care.* In their quest to deliver better care at lower costs, healthcare providers face regulatory barriers that impede the fulfillment of the triple aim—higher quality at lower cost for the entire population. Advancing a regulatory regime that is reflective of the way care will be delivered in the future is key.

- *Federal government payments will continue to increase, leading to delivery reform.* The increase of existing government payment programs, such as Medicare Advantage, coupled with the emergence of new government payment models, such as Accountable Care Organizations, will lead to delivery reform.

- *Scale matters in delivering coordinated care.* To deliver care across the continuum and to effectively manage the health of populations, scale is necessary.

Non-provider healthcare industry stakeholders have different objectives and advocate different messages than do providers to executive, legislative, and judicial branch executives at the state and federal levels. Healthcare providers must effectively communicate the necessity of scale, fewer barriers to integration, and the necessity for structuring incentives for consumers and providers to underlie delivery reform designed to deliver better care at a lower cost.

Advocacy is a critical aspect of the leadership of all healthcare organizations. Each organization will find the best way to engage governmental entities. Transformation in such a highly regulated environment will be a constant challenge.

The Customer

"Know your customer" is the watchword of today's healthcare organizations, and it is becoming increasingly important in the evolving consumer-driven market. Sophisticated and regularly conducted market research is required, since consumer preferences evolve quickly. Market intelligence about the local community will provide insights into the business-model implications of narrow networks, retail medicine, and new competitors. The market for the $n = 1$ consumers is changing, and new marketing skills will be required.

Data as the Foundation for Transformation

Most healthcare provider organizations are still managing the challenge of implementing EHRs and meeting the criteria for meaningful use. The cultural and operational challenges of implementation of this phase of digitization have been draining and often frustrating. A residency program leader recently reported that the faculty is frustrated because the change from paper to digital was slow and painful and requires more of their time; however, the residents are frustrated because digital implementation has not proceeded quickly enough and doesn't do all they want it to do.

The University of Pittsburgh Medical Center (UPMC) is a vertically integrated system engaged in population health management, for which information management has proven to be a critical success factor. Data management begins with the enrollment of the member and is tracked and accumulated during the patient's journey through the health system. Dr. Pamela Peele, one of the leading data scientists in healthcare, leads their integrated delivery and financing system innovation laboratory, which provides data-analytic tools and staff for the health plan and the delivery system.

The diverse talents of her staff include competencies in epidemiology, biostatistics, economics, statistics, physics, mathematics, and biomedical engineering. In addition, there are specific data management tools such as data visualization, data mining, financial modeling, and evaluation and predictive analytics. The data inputs are broad and include claims data from multiple sources: biometric screening, enrollment and demographic data, absenteeism data from timecards, pharmacy claims, labs, and other delivery-system data points.

The multidisciplinary approach to data management and analysis allows a focus on the individual. Through this collection of data from multiple sources, the team makes correlations to better anticipate health needs. For instance, a patient with a sole diagnosis of Parkinson's disease has a statistically predictable likelihood of requiring hospitalization. However, for a patient with a diagnosis of depression as comorbidity with Parkinson's disease, the statistical likelihood of

"When a Health Plan Knows How You Shop"
New York Times, by Natasha Singer, June 28, 2014

There may be a link between your Internet use and how often you end up in the emergency room.

At least that's one of the curious connections to emerge from a healthcare analysis project at the insurance division of the University of Pittsburgh Medical Center.

U.P.M.C. is a $12 billion nonprofit enterprise that owns hospitals in western Pennsylvania as well as a health insurance plan with about 2.4 million members. It is at the forefront of an emerging field called predictive health analytics, intended to improve patients' healthcare outcomes and contain costs. But patients themselves are often unaware of the kinds of intimate details about their households that insurers and hospitals may use to try to sway their treatment decisions.

The Pittsburgh health plan, for instance, has developed prediction models that analyze data like patient claims, prescriptions and census records to determine which members are likely to use the most emergency and urgent care, which can be expensive. Data sets of past healthcare consumption are fairly standard tools for predicting future use of health services.

But the insurer recently bolstered its forecasting models with details on members' household incomes, education levels, marital status, race or ethnicity, number of children at home, number of cars and so on. One of the sources for the consumer data U.P.M.C. used was Acxiom, a marketing analytics company that obtains consumers' information from both public records and private sources.

With the addition of these household details, the insurer turned up a few unexpected correlations: Mail-order shoppers and Internet users, for example, were likelier than some other members to use more emergency services.

continued

continued

Of course, buying furniture through, say, the Ikea catalog is unlikely to send you to the emergency-room. But it could be a proxy for other factors that do have a bearing on whether you seek urgent care, says Pamela Peele, the chief analytics officer for the U.P.M.C. insurance services division. A hypothetical patient might be a catalog shopper, for instance, because he or she is homebound or doesn't have access to transportation.

"It brings me another layer of vision, of view, that helps me figure out better prediction models and allocate our clinical resources," Dr. Peele said during a recent interview. She added: "If you are going to decrease the costs and improve the quality of care, you have to do something different."

The U.P.M.C. health plan has not yet acted on the correlations it found in the household data. But it already segments its members into different "market baskets," based on analysis of more traditional data sets. Then it assigns care coordinators to certain members flagged as high risk because they have chronic conditions that aren't being properly treated. The goal, Dr. Peele said, is for the insurer to steer those patients to primary care physicians or specialists who can provide care that is more coordinated, more consistent and less costly than sporadic emergency-room visits. The system might pinpoint, for example, high-risk asthma patients who have not yet been prescribed inhalers — and try to manage their care before they end up in emergency rooms with asthma attacks.

hospitalization increases significantly. This algorithm triggers a response from the delivery-system care management teams. Analyzing and interpreting the data means good care for the patient and money saved for the health plan. Dr. Peele is clear that she is describing an operating area for "analysis and knowledge surfacing," not an information technology function. The distinction between analytics and technology acquisition, installation, and maintenance is a bright line.

How do leaders create a data-driven organization? What is necessary technically? More importantly, what is necessary culturally? Every organization has a different level of capability. An accurate assessment of the organizational analytic capability is essential for leaders.

Many CMIOs caution that the full ability to implement the potential of the EHR and create a digitized environment takes longer than senior leaders may recognize. There are the challenges of provider data entry and interoperability of systems, as well as the inflexibility of many EHRs. Digitization is not complete with the last install of the EHR. It is likely the EHRs will be infrastructure as an entirely new digital clinical enterprise evolves. There are still many difficult technology challenges for organizations. These must be managed as the use of analytics is developed. Leaders connect all this work to the plan for the evolution of the organization to be increasingly information-driven.

Data in healthcare today has been compared to discovering the largest reserve of crude oil ever found. We don't know yet how to refine the oil into products like jet fuel, kerosene, and gasoline, but we are learning. Leaders must communicate the plan for "drilling, fracking, and refining" the data.

Collaborate Effectively

As healthcare transforms, collaboration is becoming more important. No single organization has all the required competencies or resources. Collaboration occurs at the community level as providers and local agencies work together to provide care models. Insurance companies are partnering with physicians, hospitals, health systems, and employers to provide more valuable services.

Local collaboration is imperative in providing the array of medical and social services needed for population healthcare. Collaboration that connects services such as counseling, nutrition, education, and transportation is key to the health of the population. There is a growing use of trained volunteers to serve as navigators for the health system. The navigators help with appointments, filling prescriptions, and other services that ensure the health of the patient. Collaboration involves these individuals as well as large organizations.

In many markets, provider health systems are building new and collaborative relationships with insurers. They develop mutual understanding of their individual business models, and then they address the opportunities in the market. This is a radical departure from past confrontational relationships. Nurturing and managing these relationships between payers and providers will be a key future competency. Insurers and providers understand the n = 1 expectations and must successfully collaborate to compete for the new consumer.

Health systems collaborations help achieve scale economies. Collaborative approaches to supply chain management, information technology, innovation, and other areas are increasing dramatically. Form follows function in the organizational structure of these innovative collaborations. Networks or affiliations differ in their degree of formality, and they can be self-organized or assisted by national organizations. The underlying premise is that they can be more effective in meeting the market need together rather than separately.

The evolution in information will have a profound effect on the collaboration of healthcare organizations. Collaboration in information and data management is rapidly growing. The scale necessary to fully utilize big data and predictive analytics is beyond any single organization. Cloud computing is, by definition, scalable. Exploys, Optum, and others are the beginning of new relationships driven by the opportunity to leverage: the scale of data, including the hardware to store, the software to process, and the expertise to utilize the information that healthcare is producing.

Chapter 6. Competencies:

- How will the revenue model of your organization change over the next five years? As utilization patterns change or decline, how will the operating margin of your healthcare organization be affected?

- What are your explicit plans to assume more risk? How will you outpace the competition?

- What are the differentiating features and benefits of your organization to the $n = 1$?

- What are three organizational competencies you must strengthen, while reducing expenses?

- What explicit financial and talent plans does your organization have to become a more data-driven organization?

- Have you created a linkage of your long-range financial plan to your talent management plan?

- Have you allocated enough resources and "mind share" to advocacy?

PART IV

Organizing for n = 1

We will consider organizational responses to transformation. Healthcare is composed of a multitude of different professionals dedicated to alleviating suffering and disease. Healthcare is also made up of a number of different types of organizations and industries, each acting in its own enlightened self-interest, to achieve that mission of healing.

There is not "a healthcare system" in the United States. Healthcare is provided through the interaction of a vast number of independent component parts. Any similarity of U.S. healthcare to a system is unintentional. The transformative forces now acting on healthcare are spurring innovative reorganization of these components into systems.

Over the last several decades, healthcare has been emerging from a "cottage industry" with a "mom-and-pop" organizational structure. It has become a massive business, consuming nearly a fifth of the GDP of our country. Market and regulatory forces continue to shape healthcare.

In response to the markets, healthcare reorganization has been ongoing. Part Four describes how leaders are innovatively organizing healthcare services to create competitive organizations.

Today, most healthcare organizations consider themselves successful. In spite of current success, leaders must challenge their organizational function and structure. New entrants, unencumbered by traditional structure or culture and fueled by the forces

continued

continued

of transformation, will find markets to exploit. Leading change when things are successful is a challenge. Health systems, physician groups, and others all have this challenge today. Yet leading change while things are "good" is a core leadership responsibility.

Innovation of organizational structure is occurring in every part of healthcare. Leaders are challenging the status quo. Innovation in areas such as horizontal integration, vertical integration, and adoption of new collaborative structures is widespread. Hospital systems, physicians, insurers, and industries are all innovating organizational competencies and structures in response to the market.

The true test for these organizations is in the creation of value for the consumer, the $n = 1$. Does the vertical and horizontal integration add value? Are the competencies and scale efficiencies enough to counter the dis-economies of scale in large organizations? What are the organizational features and benefits most important to the $n = 1$? Is the culture of the new organization focused on serving the individual?

Part 4 discusses organizational innovation from the standpoint of the hospital system, physician, and health plan. Each has a unique perspective. Each has unique opportunities and challenges. Their organizational innovation will be manifested in different ways. Their strategies overlap, compete, and blend with each other.

Ultimately, the $n = 1$ will determine the success of organizational innovation.

"Does the $n = 1$, the unique individual consumer, want to buy what you have created?"

CHAPTER 7

Integrated Health Systems

Hospitals and health systems are a product of their geography, mission, heritage, culture, and environment. Their historic core business is the hospital. Following two waves of consolidation since 1990, most of the nation's 5,000 community hospitals are owned or operated by a multi-hospital system.[30]

Approximately 4,000 of the 5,000 community hospitals in the nation are not-for-profit; the remainder are investor-owned. The not-for-profits stated goals and covenants are to serve the needs of their local communities. Investor-owned health systems serve community needs and other goals as required by their shareholders. The fact remains that, for all the diversity of health systems, there is commonality of strategies, which occurs in part because of the similarity in community needs. The financial and regulatory direction of payers, both governmental and commercial, is also similar. The entire industry is heavily regulated by other organizations such as the Joint Commission.

Hospitals have aggressively pursued horizontal integration for the past twenty-five years. Creation of integrated delivery systems has been in response to the local markets. These health systems have created innovative organizational designs to meet the unique needs of their communities. They have pursued horizontal integration with other hospital providers. Most integrated systems have also pursued vertical integration strategies with physicians, health plans, home-health, and other related health services.

Chapter 7 will examine vertical and horizontal integration from the perspective of a hospital-based health system. Organizational innovation is blurring the boundaries between health system, physician group, and health plan. This trend will continue to accelerate as the market demands higher value for healthcare services. The organizational innovation of creating a system where none currently exists is the value added.

Horizontal Integration

For most of the 1900s, hospitals were highly fragmented, prideful, and autonomous, with a horizon only as far as their own geography. Most hospitals were governed by local leaders and contained physicians focused on that specific institution. The earliest multi-hospital systems were often aggregations of separate institutions created by faith-based sponsors to serve different communities. Systems were created because of the need for the sponsors to consolidate their oversight, often because the systems grew and the sponsor's numbers diminished.

Hospital leaders of thirty to forty years ago saw how consolidation of multiple hospitals could increase capital available for technology and growth, increase the talent pool, and allow the development of clinical standards that diminished variation of medical care. Hospital and health system leaders demonstrated the value of health systems to initially skeptical hospital boards and physicians.

Horizontal integration, whether in the hospital or other industries, focuses on creating scale economies, market synergies, and information sharing. These efficiencies achieve a lower cost of production and enhanced market position. Horizontal integration can be particularly effective in capital-intense industries such as hospitals. Our research has found that there are four primary areas of efficiency that can be gained through horizontal integration of hospitals:

- *Scale economies,* such as supply purchasing and management of investments;

- *Shared resources,* such as financial, human resources and legal services, strategic planning;

- *Shared infrastructure,* such as an information technology platform;

- *Learning organization,* including shared knowledge and talent acquisition.

Identification of specific, tangible and relevant goals for integration is critical to success. Not all the goals achieved through horizontal integration require full merger or acquisition into health systems with common ownership. For example, group purchasing organizations like VHA, Premier, MedAssets, and many others have created horizontally integrated groups of healthcare organizations with the goal of more efficient group purchasing.

There are lessons to be learned from horizontal integration in other industries—for example, commercial banking. Similarities between health systems and commercial banking include a requirement for consumer-specific data, which that must be private and accurate; a high degree of government regulation; a capital (e.g., buildings)-intensive business model; the importance of technology (ATM to banking and radiology equipment for hospitals); and local presence.

Both industries have scale opportunities. The first lesson from banking leaders is that consolidation isn't as easy as it looks. Projections are frequently optimistic or overstated. Banking consolidation, as in healthcare, highlights the challenges not only of different corporate cultures, but also of different geographies. In addition, business challenges such as integrating information systems in a timely way are similar. Lastly, many customers may feel grateful for the advantages gained through consolidation, but others will move their business because some feature or benefit has been "consolidated out of" their legacy bank.

When organizations are considering horizontal integration, a clear agreement on future vision is important. What is the shared understanding of the n = 1, retail markets, and population health? How will integration assist in digitization and leveraging the disruptive scientific innovation? The horizontal integration must be based on the market of the future.

Early and candid discussions between prospective merger partners will pay dividends. Agreement on goals and objectives, although important, is frequently illusive. For instance it might be troublesome if one party believes that theirs is the single management system that will prevail following the merger, while the other party believes that there will be due diligence as to which management system prevails. It is easy to predict conflict and a poor outcome. These are difficult conversations, particularly in community-based not-for-profit healthcare organizations. Many times it is the community boards that have differing interpretations of community need and how to best meet it.

Needless to say there are legal and political considerations galore in all of these discussions.

Larger health systems, with more experience in horizontal integration, will have a well-defined integration model. This may result in less flexibility but higher success for new partners. Health systems that are new to horizontal integration may have more opportunity for trial and error in determining the best synergies with prospective partners. Execution of strategies around scale and shared resources are generally measurable and discrete. They depend on executive support, talented management, and clear goals and objectives. Vision and strategies are interesting and important, but execution is mandatory.

Over-optimism for the creation of synergistic value is one major pitfall to successful outcomes from horizontal integration. Often leaders planning the integration have a bias for the ability of the system to create value in centralization, consolidation, or integration. This bias comes from their perspective as system leaders responsible for system-created value. Leaders operating closer to the "front-line action" or patients may have a different bias as to the value created by centralization. Assessments of what is possible, or even what is the desired outcome, are dramatically influenced by the leader's position in the organization. Success in integration depends on the productive resolution of the bias conflicts.[31] The single most important key to success in achieving synergy is "sizing the prize." Rigorous and objective measurements of synergy must be identified as well as specific accountability for key performance indicators demonstrating its accomplishment. When leaders create specific and objective measures, the danger of bias can be mitigated.

Healthcare is a knowledge-based profession and industry. As market pressure continues to grow and payment systems evolve, health systems that *learn faster* and *implement effectively* have a significant advantage. Early in the process, partners in horizontal integration should develop a shared vision for the learning organization resulting from the integration. Sharing the scale opportunities of group purchasing, creating a contracting network, and sharing administrative costs will not be enough in the future. This vision for a learning organization is often what will inspire and gain the support of clinicians.

The term "learning organization" refers to an organization that is committed to transformation and development of its employees. Organizations in highly competitive and transforming industries, such as consulting, technology, and healthcare, find success as learning organizations. Peter Senge notes that a learning organization has five main features: systems thinking, personal mastery, mental models, shared vision, and team learning.[32]

In any industry, horizontal integration can give rise to fears of price increases as markets consolidate. Competition usually resolves those concerns. In the case of consolidating hospitals, the payment and regulatory structure seems to influence prices more than consolidation. This is an area of significant study and debate among academics.[33] Consolidation of physicians and health insurers gives rise to similar concerns. The legal and regulatory environment is nebulous, but the market forces driving consolidation are clear and unrelenting.

Many, if not most, markets will have healthcare organizations struggling to survive. These organizations may be important to the community and may not have many options. Mergers, consolidation, acquisitions, affiliations, or other forms of integration with others, either in their community or outside, may be the best choice. The balance between the concern of market consolidation and demonstrated value will be important. Boards, policy makers, politicians, and regulators will all have their opinions.

Today's unrelenting transformative forces require organizational innovation. What if, in the future, digitization and democratization of healthcare information can inexpensively create efficiencies that today horizontal integration creates via expensive and complex organizational structure? Do the barriers to entry into healthcare provision diminish? Does disintegration and customization of health services become possible? What is being learned from other industries? The key guiding principle is that *the only constant is change.*

Leaders must keep looking ahead and asking needed questions. Future organizational innovation may look very different from today's.

Vertical Integration

Vertical integration by hospital systems refers to formal ownership relationships with physician groups or health insurance plans. This chapter will not discuss hospital integration into services such as supply chain management or revenue cycle management. This so-called backward integration may be a valuable tool for lowering administrative costs.

Vertical integration is a strategy deployed by hospital systems for decades. Ownership of health plans by hospital systems has waxed and waned since the early 1980s. Physician employment and integration have followed similar patterns. These strategies are directed at improving the continuum of care and producing value for the consumer. As noted previously, healthcare is not a system. Vertical integration creates alignment of incentives and a deployment of resources to create a system of care.

Most hospital systems are vertically integrating with physicians, and many are aligning with health plans in innovative ways. Each market will determine the pace and the value of vertical integration. The imperative of meeting the market's needs was one of the major lessons of past vertical integration efforts. Understanding the market and its dynamics is important. Hospital systems moving prematurely or misinterpreting market signals can encounter significant problems. Vertical integration is neither cheap nor easy.

Even hospital systems that have decades of experience with vertical integration may receive only 30 percent of their total revenue through their vertically integrated market channels. For the remainder of their revenue, they depend on health plans and physicians with whom they compete. The hospital system's timeline, market position, and expectations of the economics of vertical integration are important considerations.

Opportunities of vertical integration include:

- Higher value of the delivery system continuum of care
- Service delivery difficult for competitors to replicate
- Higher barrier to entry
- Market intelligence
- New products and services
- Knowledge transfer
- Broader and richer data and information

Challenges of vertical integration include:

- Competition with existing customers
- Lack of industry-specific expertise
- Management of an "internal economy"
- Integration of differing financial models
- Different customers for each component of the system

Most markets are stimulating healthcare organizations to pursue vertical integration. Vertical integration may be via ownership or as a component of another organization's virtually integrated system. The system performance required to provide value to n = 1 will determine when and how vertical integration is useful. As was noted earlier, healthcare today is not a system, but, to bring value to n = 1, a system must be created.

"Apprehensive, Many Doctors Shift to Jobs
with Salaries"
New York Times, by Elisabeth Rosenthal, February 13, 2014

In 2013, 64 percent of job offers filled through Merritt Hawkins, one of the nation's leading physician placement firms, involved hospital employment, compared with only 11 percent in 2004. The firm anticipates a rise to 75 percent in the next two years.

Today, about 60 percent of family doctors and pediatricians, 50 percent of surgeons, and 25 percent of surgical subspecialists—such as ophthalmologists and ear, nose, and throat surgeons—are employees rather than independent, according to the American Medical Association. "We're seeing it changing fast," said Mark E. Smith, president of Merritt Hawkins.

Vertical Integration with Physicians

The history of vertical integration of health systems with physicians has ebbed and flowed over the last fifty years. Many specialists closely tied to hospital procedures, such as radiologists and anesthesiologists, have been employed by hospitals since the 1970s. In the 1980s, intensivists, physicians specializing in treating patients in intensive care units, became more common.

During the late 1980s and early 1990s, active discussion of

healthcare reform generated interest in provider-owned-and-sponsored health plans. In addition, primary care and certain high-volume specialty physicians were employed by hospitals in anticipation of capitated payment models. After healthcare reform failed in the mid-1990s, many of the integration efforts between hospitals, health plans, and physicians were painfully terminated. In some markets, vertical integration continued as a viable strategy. Many difficult lessons were learned from those vertical integration efforts. Organizations that persevered in their vertical integration strategies gained significant experience.

Over the last decade, many health systems employed primary care physicians to build distribution channels for patients to the hospital and to specialists, and to provide consistent value throughout the continuum of care. In addition, the economics of primary care and certain specialty practices has become much less attractive, resulting in many physicians seeking employment with hospital systems. So there are many strategic reasons for hospitals and health systems to be in an active growth mode with physician practices.

The likelihood of success of vertical integration strategies with physicians is greatly increased if there is a shared vision. Many times, pragmatic considerations take precedence, e.g., a defensive strategy to prevent key physicians from leaving the health system or the community, or maintaining hospital inpatient revenue by ensuring the right mixes of physicians. Often a hospital executive, who historically viewed physicians as customers, is in charge of physician strategy, including compensation and business model. The required shift in mental models and relationships can be challenging for all involved.

Vertical integration of hospital systems with physicians is a high-risk and difficult strategy, but imperative for future success. Trust and vision are required. Examples of value realized from health systems and physicians jointly working together with similar vision and objectives are:

- Development of new products and services,
- New branding opportunities for vertically integrated services

that can be marketed to existing or new customers,
- Enhanced information-sharing between the components of the vertically integrated system,
- Identification of key performance expectations in clinical and service areas,
- Attracting and retaining high-quality professionals.

Michael Porter believes the "value chain" creates the integration opportunity.[34] In his view, each component of an integrated system can add value to a customer. Each intersection between components can subtract value. The organization should specify and quantify the opportunity for value creation for each component. In addition, with each opportunity for customer value, there is a corresponding potential for value loss. The potential value creation and loss should be clearly identified and quantified. As the health system pursues a strategy of vertical integration, creation of customer value gain and value loss can be measured. Examples of lost value include:

- Loss of physician productivity due to changed incentives, bureaucracy, and new information technology;
- Real and perceived competition with other physician groups not employed by the health system;
- Patient perception of reduction of choice of physicians;
- Increasing costs of managing physician practices within a health system.

Vertical integration of a hospital system with physicians must produce overall net value for the consumer. This can be created at the individual physician group level, at the level of the entire system, or with innovative new service offerings (population health or retail services). Each specialty will have different opportunities for value creation with consumers. While understanding the consumer's needs is critical, one key to value production for consumers is a satisfying practice environment for the physicians. A sustainable, successful business will produce the most satisfying practice environment for physicians.

If physicians are frustrated in the integrated system, patient satisfaction is likely to suffer.

Disparate incentives create challenges for successful hospital-physician vertical integration. A shared vision for a sustainable and successful business is difficult to achieve. The hospital executive's incentive may be to preserve the traditional hospital business. Physicians are trying to create personal economic stability and predictability for their practice. Both parties may be seeking insulation and stability rather than innovation in a new business. The lack of common vision can lead physicians to develop an "employee mentality," while the hospital leaders are focused on the "subsidies" being paid to the physician group. In these instances a *transactional relationship* is forged rather than a transformational relationship.

Transactional relationships are defined solely by the terms and conditions of employment and the compensation arrangements. In these relationships, there is no incentive for transformation or shared vision. It is solely about the hospital "owning" the physicians and the physicians being "employees." Transactional relationships frequently begin to unravel as soon as the deal is closed. There are few greater management challenges than a previously independent, highly trained physician now in a transactional relationship. The transactional relationship is always subject to interpretation by all parties. The specifics of the contract guide all matters. When there is a difference between expectation and reality, there is frustration and conflict.

A transformative relationship is based on professional relationships within the medical group. The professional self-management and accountability within the group is crucial to meeting the challenges of the future. Even in long-standing medical groups this dynamic takes constant effort to maintain. The culture, relationships, and peer pressure keep the group aligned and moving forward.

The conversion of transactional relationships to transformative relationships will be critically important for hospital systems. Development of physician leaders is imperative. These leaders create sustainable and innovative business models within their medical groups.

There are many outstanding health system medical groups that have developed the management and leadership infrastructure necessary for transformation. The Cleveland Clinic and the Mayo Clinic have had decades to evolve. Newly created health system-based physician groups will need to mature and evolve rapidly to keep up with transformation of healthcare. Learning from other medical groups is key.

Health system vertical integration into health insurance is an important requirement in the transforming healthcare industry. Vertical integration strategy into insurance is often verbalized as:

- "We want to move upstream to gain part or all of the premium dollar."
- "We need to control the distribution of the premium."
- "We believe that we can perform administrative functions less expensively than health insurance companies."
- "We control care management, and the value created by health insurance companies is diminished with healthcare reform."

"When Hospital Systems Buy Health Insurers"
New York Times, by Austin Frakt, May 25, 2014

There are several reasons hospitals might want to be in the insurance business, or more closely aligned with insurers. By acting in cooperation, a unified organization might be able to better design incentives for higher-quality care. Or, by combining similar functions like human resources or tech support, the organization might cut costs. A joint provider-insurer may also be better able to adapt to—and make more money from—new Medicare payment models in the Affordable Care Act. Eventually, an organization that combines the functions of healthcare provision and healthcare insurance might have a leg up in the market, putting competitors at a disadvantage or driving them out.

Vertical Integration with Health Insurance

There is a growing rationale for providers becoming involved in the health insurance business. The Blue Cross Blue Shield organization has its heritage in the hospital business dating to the early 1930s and the Depression. As far back as the mid-1800s, the Sisters of Providence began a prepaid health insurance scheme with miners in the Northwest. Most of the largest 100 health systems in the country have a health plan.

In the 1980s and early 1990s, it was common for large hospitals and health systems to develop and operate HMOs. Many of the health system-owned health plans were sold. HMOs lost their luster. However, there are prominent examples, such as Intermountain Healthcare, Sentara, and Providence Health and Services, that have maintained and grown their health plans. Many larger health systems that do not operate health plans are exploring that option in response to the market.

Transference of risk to the consumer and providers leads health systems to consider vertically integrating into health insurance. Regulatory changes, emanating from the ACA, have limited the health insurer's actuarial, underwriting, and marketing tools. Future value will be the ability to price risk at a profitable level, then manage that risk through sophisticated clinical systems, information, consumer engagement, and incentives. Health systems have an opportunity to design sophisticated clinical systems that can best manage risk. They must employ or have relationships with professionals competent in managing a health insurance infrastructure.

Management of an insured population over time is a very different task than running a healthcare delivery organization or a medical group. Large health systems experienced in managing risk have found their focus must be across the continuum of care. The nature of the problems and conflicts when the provider and consumer are assuming risk are very different than the fee-for-service model of healthcare.

When the health system "controls the premium dollar," an internal economy within the health system is created as dollars are distributed to those providing services. The contentious meetings regarding issues such as "fair payment principles" or reimbursement levels for hospitals or doctors from their own health plan reflect the fact that controlling the premium dollar creates a new set of challenges. However, there are important opportunities to change incentives for providers and patients and to test innovative new ways of caring for people.

Every provider-owned health plan holds meetings where the health plan leader presents the customer's expectations for the premium. The hospital and physician leaders need enough of the "medical cost" in the premium to support the demands of their provider constituents. The leaders may have personal performance incentives attached to the success of their discrete business unit. The health plan must set an expectation of continual reduction in the healthcare expense trend. The system must grow the plan for it to be administratively efficient and actuarially sound. That requires a competitive premium. Remember, if there is waste taken out of the system, then the system must grow its customer base to support operations. This is the internal economy to be managed in provider-owned health plans.

As with all vertical integration strategies, it's absolutely key to attract and retain knowledgeable talent. In the case of health systems integrating with health insurers, that means attracting talent with experience and understanding of the health insurance industry. These leaders must also possess the cultural flexibility to operate in both the provider and the health insurance worlds. Skeptics of provider-owned health plans point out that success will be measured by the willingness for creative destruction of the core business, the hospital. As most leaders in health systems have a heritage in hospitals, the skeptics believe that the push-pull of cultures in a hospital system-owned health plan causes the health system executives to bend to the provider perspective.

Just as the aspiration for horizontal integration is to create a learning organization, vertical integration into health insurance enhances organizational learning. The insurance function deals face-to-face with paying customers, while the health system historically has been paid by the health insurer acting as intermediary between the provider and the customer. Customers have expectations and requirements in a provider-owned health plan, and these preferences and demands can be articulated directly to the delivery system, rather than through a "provider relations specialist" from an insurer.

Understanding the perspective of the consumer through the eyes of the health plan is increasingly important. This is the best opportunity for the health system to understand the needs of the n = 1 consumer. The intimate, face-to-face consumer relationship is important as health-benefit decisions involving networks of care are made. In the future, many healthcare organizations will be seeking a direct relationship with the consumer. Health systems will be at risk of disintermediation.

Here are two examples of how the providers can identify and adopt new programs with information gathered from their health plan:

- The health plan of a large health system, in dialogue with a local employer, determined that productivity and time away from the workplace were key employer concerns. The health system installed a telemedicine kiosk that enabled employees, confidentially, to gain health evaluations and screening via the telemedicine team. Later, the health system was able to determine if on-site providers made sense for the employer. Productive time for the employees increased; the employer was pleased.
- A provider-sponsored health plan analyzed claims data from an employer and identified the need for enhanced prenatal care. The health system was able to place providers and programs to assist in prenatal care to decrease high-cost preterm deliveries.

When the health system looks beyond its boundaries of delivering care into the customer world of employer, patient, or government, it has the opportunity to innovate and create value. The opportunity to shape incentives and match them with healthcare services is key to successful vertical integration with insurance. The challenge for providers is the reduction in revenue resulting from more efficient care processes. These programs impact the traditional revenue of the system. The programs could be high-risk pregnancy prevention, low-intensity low back pain treatment, or others.

The employer community is unsympathetic to this issue. When asked about sharing savings resulting from more efficient care process, an Intel executive was clear: "You have been caring for our employees with a broken system and charging us for it. We are not paying you because you are beginning to fix your system. Our executives improve process all the time that lowers our revenue, and our customers don't care. You get no sympathy and certainly no cost sharing from us."

There is a growing blurring of the boundaries between health insurers and providers. Providers are becoming more like health insurers, and health insurers are developing competencies of providers. Organizations will decide to build, buy, or partner. New arrangements between insurers and providers are emerging, using the skills and competencies of each to maximize the value proposition for the n = 1 consumer. Skilled leaders who have respect and understanding for the different worlds of delivery and insurance will be pivotal in collaboration. The fact that WellPoint chose Joseph R. Swedish, an experienced health system leader, as its CEO[35] is indicative of the merging of the provider and health insurance worlds. Mr. Swedish's knowledge of the provider world has facilitated new types of collaboration to bring value to the n =1.

Chapter 7. Integrated Healthcare:

- What are your organization's beliefs, stories, and mental models regarding the value of horizontal and vertical integration? Which are helpful, and which are not? What needs to change?

- What are the three most important lessons from vertical integration in your organization? How has it changed the organization?

- Rate the various physician relationships of the health system as transactional or transformational. What difference will this make?

- If the health system has a health plan, what is the long-term strategic plan? How big must it become? How soon? Why?

- If the health system does not have a health plan, what is the plan to profit from taking and managing risk for populations? What is the long-term plan?

CHAPTER 8

Physicians

What was once a cottage industry of physician practice has been evolving toward a more "corporate and scalable" practice for fifty years. The pace of change has stepped up in the last decade. As with every aspect of healthcare, this plays out differently in every community.

Profound forces are impacting physicians' professional lives. The economic challenges to physician practices are well documented. The administrative expense, insurance rules, and regulatory compliance issues are at the core of the change. The need to change the practice is not just about the economic realities.

The healing relationship between a physician and a patient is being changed by a number of factors. A patient's ability to access information about her own health—the democratization of information—alters the healing relationship. Patients accessing information about physician quality redefines the physician-patient relationship. Increased financial responsibility of patients for their healthcare will also have an impact on their relationship to their physician.

This democratization of information, commonly known as transparency, will continue to alter the professional practice of physicians. The leveling of access to information between patient and physician is fundamental to the transformation.

The experience of other industries shows us that the current gap in reliable information about provider quality will be filled. The information may not be perfect, but it will be good enough. The market will continue to push transparency. The n = 1 will demand it.

Digitization creates opportunities for physicians to use analytics within their specialties to identify opportunities. Analytics improving clinical process are important and can provide a competitive advantage.

Physicians are creating innovative organizational structures to serve patient expectations. Physicians are integrating with other physicians and other healthcare organizations. These organizations have several desired outcomes:

- Infrastructure support, capital, and information technology;
- Market-driven payment models, such as ACOs;
- Creation of new clinical products and services;
- Recruiting and retaining of physicians.

Physicians, by the nature of the profession, may have personal goals beyond those of their organization. The physician's personal goals may include financial security, "cash-out" of partners in medical groups, reduction of administrative responsibilities, and many others. Physicians will have their own rationales for integration.

These goals can create a platform for success. Medical groups, whether they are independent or part of a health system, must be responsive to consumers. Providing exceptional medical care is the measure that matters. Medical groups that are innovative learning organizations are the most likely to succeed. Medical groups understand that the n = 1 consumer creates the definition of "exceptional medical care." As we have discussed, different people will have different expectations. A medical group will create an experience for the patient with a broad perception of exceptional medical care.

Learning organizations continuously transform, which keeps them competitive. The cardiovascular program director of a large health system recently described a meeting where 200 cardiologists, cardiovascular surgeons, and administrative and clinical support teams gathered to identify the areas of system focus for clinical improvement, standardization, and innovation. There was excitement as they shared their leading practices and insights about how to work with their colleagues to advance clinical care processes. They had painstakingly developed a culture of data-driven clinical care across their practices. Enthusiasm was expressed about the use of predictive analytics tools to identify areas for improvement and quantify the impact of clinical changes. The leaders in this meeting represented hundreds of other cardiovascular clinicians across thirty-five hospitals in five states. They understood the importance of their opportunity. This "expert-to-expert" collaboration is the hallmark of a learning organization.

Not long ago, it would have been difficult to get any one of these groups to talk to each other, since they were solely focused on their individual practices. Physicians may have been intellectually curious, but they did not have the vision or the tools to effectively collaborate with other experts. Today, physician leadership has been enabled by digitization and the resulting analysis of information. The consensus is that there will now be an acceleration of their agenda for cost-effective, high-quality care. Through expert-to-expert (E2E) collaboration, physicians are identifying ways they can create high-performance learning organizations that will make their practices successful in the future.

The structure of medical practice has changed dramatically over the last decade. More physicians are opting for employment models, either with medical groups or with health systems. In a 2013 survey conducted by Jackson Healthcare,[36] a healthcare staffing company polled 3,456 physicians. When asked which form of employment they chose, respondents reported the following:

- Employed by a hospital–26 percent, up 6 percent from 2012;
- Ownership stake in a practice–22 percent, down 1 percent from 2012;
- Solo practice–15 percent, down 6 percent from 2012;
- Works for physician-owned practice, but has no ownership stake–15 percent, up 3 percent from 2012;
- Employed by physician practice that is owned by a hospital or health system–14 percent, down 1 percent from 2012;
- Independent contractor–8 percent, down 1 percent from 2012.

There are many models of clinical integration, contracting, and information sharing. They are often unique and circumstance-specific, but attempt to serve the needs of the market and patients. They include ACO, IPA, alliances, and practice affiliations. The diversity of these relationships is remarkable.

It's very difficult to know whether we will have too many or too few physicians in the future. What is certain is the lag of at least seven years to either increase or decrease the number of clinicians coming through training programs. Consequently, for the next decade, the number of new physicians coming into healthcare will be roughly the same. As the 80 million baby boomers reach the age when they will use more health services, and as the ACA and Medicaid expansion programs provide coverage to previously uncovered individuals, there will be an increased demand for physicians. Balancing the increased demand will be the use of other providers, innovations, and changes in care processes. The phrase "practicing at the top of your license" describes how the physician's expertise will increasingly be used. Physician expertise must be used effectively.

Transformational forces will impact physicians of different specialties in different ways. The forces of n = 1, digitization, and disruptive innovation will require physicians of different specialties to consider different structural models to support their practices. These transformational forces will change the nature of what they do, where it's done, with whom they compete, and the incentives that drive them.

Primary Care Physicians

The transformational forces of healthcare are creating a dynamic future for primary care physicians. They will have many new tools to help manage their patients more efficiently and effectively. As the data above demonstrates, primary care physicians have consolidated more than any other physicians. They have joined large organizations like multi-specialty groups and health systems. From a strategic stand-point, large organizations have considered the primary care physicians as a "distribution channel" for specialty physicians or hospital and "fishing net" for fee-for-service patients.

As the transformational forces grow, we are seeing primary care strategies built around the transference of risk either to populations or to unique individuals. Primary care physicians are actively pursuing one or both of those strategies in many markets. For example, the "direct primary care" or "concierge" practices focus on individuals who desire greater access and more personalized care and who are willing to pay. In general, the direct primary care practice charges each consumer a membership fee and, in exchange, provides customized health services.

These concierge practices are estimated to have grown from approximately 800 physicians in 2010 to 5,000 physicians in 2014.[37] Some practices are all-concierge, and some have partial concierge practices. This model continues to be refined and may gain importance as healthcare continues its transformation.

Other primary care physicians are creating healthcare homes, often in association with larger health systems or insurers. These practices may participate in population-based healthcare models as well as fee-for-service models. In the healthcare home, digitization, mobile devices, and innovation make team medicine possible. Healthcare homes will continue to evolve and become more sophisticated over time. The setting, particularly in conjunction with other providers, is ideal for further digitization and predictive analytics in a population-based model.

Thus, primary care should no longer be considered as only a distribution channel, but as the interface between the consumer and the health system. The vast majority of patient healthcare interactions occur with primary care physicians or clinical teams.

Medical groups and health systems understand that the frequent patient encounters, or "touches," that occur in primary and community-based care strongly influence how the consumer views the brand. In retail healthcare, this equity created in the healthcare brand is of critical importance. Primary care physicians and their teams provide the first and largest impression of the brand. Branded "closeness to the customer" will be increasingly important and contested as new entrants enter the market.

The new entrants into the primary care provider space, such as retail pharmacies, retail clinics, or health insurance-sponsored care sites, will be establishing closeness to the customer and creating brand awareness. Historically, patients have selected individual physicians when they decide on care. The propagation of medical groups, the "corporatization" of medicine, narrow networks, and the increasing brand consciousness of the public make branding of comprehensive primary care services critically important. Given more attention to price, convenience, and satisfaction, consumers may be more likely to select a brand than an individual physician. Narrow networks with appealing features and benefits and with a trusted brand will be many consumers' choice.

Specialty Physicians

What incisive questions should specialty physicians be asking? Many of the strategic questions for specialty physicians are grounded in the n = 1 of consumerism. Now more financially accountable, consumers have more information about physician pricing, quality, and treatment options. How availability of information will affect consumer behavior will vary person-to-person, market-by-market, and physician-to-physician. It is a trend that is just beginning.

The high cost and complexity of specialty services creates an opportunity for marketing specialty services across broader markets. The ready access to information creates a national and, to a lesser extent, global market. Competition is becoming more acute for specialty services in larger urban areas and nationally between large national health systems, such as the Cleveland Clinic and the Mayo Clinic. Using monetary incentives to encourage patients to visit a "center of excellence" is likely to continue to grow. From an employer standpoint, the center of excellence may be less expensive than local options for complex clinical issues. It may also have a national brand, thus increasing employee acceptance. Lastly, it might carry the perception, if not the reality, of higher quality.

Most specialty physicians will have the opportunity to be part of medical groups and networks of physicians that participate in population-based health plans. In this setting, the medical group or health system receives a budgeted payment to care for a population over a period of time. The role of the specialty physician is to provide a timely, cost-effective service as requested: no more care than needed, no less. The successful medical groups managing risk have high levels of control and oversight over high-cost specialty services. The specialists engaged in these networks will be committed to the overarching goal of cost-effective, high-quality care for the covered population.

The majority of specialty programs are not neatly bifurcated into high-intensity, high-value specialty services and population healthcare specialty services. One key strategic question for specialty physicians is, Can you practice as a nationally competitive "super specialist" while working as a part of the population health team? Given the importance of the question, it is worthwhile for a specialty physician, medical group, and health system to discuss how consumers are likely to be segmented.

Important topics for questions by specialty physicians, medical groups, and health systems are:

- How to price specialty services (e.g. high-priced premium, high-value, or low-cost)
- How to brand the specialty service for a national market or part of an integrated local product or both
- Positioning the practice for talented new physicians. For example, is there a need for physicians who want a specific practice environment for research? Talent needs will follow the strategy.
- What are the implications of participating in both premium "super specialty" and population health specialty services, and what requirements do each demand?

Specialist services are going to be influenced not only by increasing information available to consumers and changing market incentives, but also by digitization and disruptive innovation. Specialists have been adapting to new treatment methodologies throughout their careers. The amount of data and information available will be a game-changer. The automation of medical records, sensors, monitors, and mobile devices are creating a tsunami of data and information that will change the nature of specialty practices.

Specialty physician leaders must focus on the consumer market. Successful specialists will be aware of competitive new entrants with new opportunities to serve consumers. Physician leaders will create comfort and energy for change within the specialty physician group.

Radiology and laboratory services are two specialty areas that have significantly transformed. They are both highly technology dependent and have been digitized earlier than most other areas of medicine. These specialties will change as the influence of digitization, automation, and predictive analytics continues to accelerate. These specialties are not only highly information- and technology-dependent; they are also scalable. There has been, and will continue to be, rapid consolidation. The opportunities arising from the digitization, large data-bases, sensors, and analytics are tremendously exciting. Radiology and laboratory services are worth keeping an eye on because these specialties foreshadow changes in other specialties.

Physician Groups

Primary care and specialty physicians practice in a multitude of settings. Medical groups such as the Mayo Clinic and the Cleveland Clinic have long histories as multi-specialty groups with strong cultures. Their sophistication as centers of team medicine, research, and medical education are well described. There are many other medical groups that have achieved high levels of excellence in population health. The Kaiser Permanente Medical Group has served the Kaiser Health Plan for many decades. HealthCare Partners, a multispecialty medical group and physician network originating in California, has been perfecting population-based healthcare and has been taking capitation payments for decades.

The mission of these medical groups may be different, but physician leadership is the common thread. These groups capitalize on opportunities created by the transformational forces of the future because they have a collegial and transformational rather than a transactional physician group culture.

Only a minority of physicians practice in well-established multi-specialty group practice today. Dr. Toby Cosgrove has predicted that many more physicians will join large group-practice corporate models with salaries, performance reviews, team medicine, and scale economics.[38] Physicians choose their practice setting based on personal beliefs, experiences, and preferences. Physician expectations for lifestyle and workload are frequently based on what were the prevailing models of practice when they started. For example, physicians who entered practice when the prevailing mode was independent specialty may view the future differently than physicians who are entering practice today, when the employment model prevails.

Physicians with decades in practice are now immersed in rapid transformation. They are seeing a change to their profession that many do not understand and certainly did not anticipate. They may feel they dedicated their lives to a profession that promised autonomy, service to patients, and the resulting rewards. They may feel that a covenant has been broken. Certainly, other industries have undergone dramatic change, and professionals in those industries have faced similar challenges. But the physician profession is unique, personal, and sacred. Sensitivity and understanding to these feelings by physician and health system leaders may benefit change management.

How do health systems and physicians who have vertically integrated create a culture, physician leadership, management, and incentive structure for successful transformation? Well-established multi-specialty group practices have decades of experience and deep culture, and yet they know that they too will be challenged.[39] The current pace of transformation suggests that newly formed physician groups will not have decades to develop the culture or the management and leadership systems.

Physicians can be frustrated and emotional about the impact of transformational change. The change, even if seemingly positive, impacts their professional lives and their patients in ways they can't control. For example, most physicians agree that the implementation of EHR allows better patient care, but the inefficiency of data entry is frustrating and beyond the control of physicians. The loss of control and interference with their care of the patient can generate skepticism as to the value of the change. Leadership is required to resolve the issues.

The future is likely to involve payment changes, increased challenges to physician autonomy, and other "hot-button" issues. As healthcare change continues, the relationship between medical groups, health systems, and their physicians is likely to be increasingly challenging, and healthcare organizations must plan for this.

Most physicians spend their lives providing the best possible care for their patients. They may not spend a great deal of energy understanding the transformation occurring around them. They may experience changes that can make it more difficult, rather than easier, to care for their patients.

Patients have different expectations regarding information and control of their care. This alteration in the historic healing relationship and the sacred trust can be very difficult to accept. Some physicians will find these changes very difficult, while others will welcome the opportunity to work with their patients in different ways.

The difference between their mental model of professional reality and how they are actually living it creates frustration. It makes no difference whether it's a health system or a medical group: leadership must understand and attempt to ameliorate the frustration. This begins with providing an inspiring vision of the future. Leadership must demonstrate commitment to that vision, not just words.

Physician leadership, physician education, and communication are required. Conversations with CEOs and healthcare leaders of all types support the importance of developing a physician organization with strong leadership and a followership educated in the transformations occurring in healthcare.

Leaders must ask difficult questions. They must also listen to difficult questions. Only through the give and take of questioning can the balance between the concerns of physicians and transformational forces be achieved. Not all questions will have answers. Many times the only response to a question is a set of choices. If physicians are openly engaged in the discussion, they may understand that there is not an answer but only a choice. It is not uncommon in medicine to not have an absolute answer, but only a series of choices. People can appreciate and accept the results when they are involved in the discussion of the choices.

Each physician organization must develop its own culture of inquiry. How an organization engages in questioning, whom it engages in inquiry, the tenor of the conversations, and other elements are unique to each organization. The key is to make asking questions part of the culture. Be vulnerable, be courageous, and engage your colleagues. Be respectful of all involved. Trust the process of inquiry. Always remember what you are all about, your healing mission.

Chapter 8. Physicians:

- What are three ways the physician organization will be different in three years? Why is that change important? Who needs to participate in the change?

- Where are the transformational forces of digitization and scientific innovation impacting physician specialties? How will consumers react? What are physicians' options?

- Although it is seemingly impossible, how would someone perform a specific clinical activity at 70 percent of the cost, in a way that's more convenient for the patient, and with demonstrably better quality? Who would be the new entrant who would do that? What would be the enabling technology, which may not exist today?

CHAPTER 9

Health Insurers

The world of health insurance has changed dramatically over the last several years. The impact of the ACA is profound and continues to evolve. The n = 1 consumer, digitization, and disruptive innovation have profoundly changed insurers.

Health insurers have increasing business from the government. WellPoint, in a recent statement, reported that government program contribution constituted 45 percent of their total revenue in 2013, an increase from 10 percent just a few years ago. The individual market is of prime importance for all health insurers. WellPoint's research[40] revealed the following individual priorities in choosing health insurance plans:

- Low price
- Brand
- Provider network

Insurers are seeking relationships with providers that give them affordability and quality. Relationships to accept payment for value are important. Insurers continue to leverage their size in return for volume and payment discounts. They are innovating with new network structures and incentives. Insurers aspire to develop trust and true partnerships with key providers.

Insurers are developing different strategies depending on the product, geography, provider relationships, and their product penetration (density). These can include but are not limited to:

- ACOs
- Centers of excellence
- Staff-model delivery
- Patient-centered healthcare homes
- Aligned incentive schemes with payment for healthcare trend reduction and quality scores
- Vertical integration into medical groups and health systems through insurer ownership
- Risk-sharing arrangements and capitalization of multi-specialty medical groups

The level of creativity and innovation in provider network management is extremely high. Jay Gellert, CEO of Health Net, recently stated, "Tailored networks are the key for insurers. The consumer can decide which network makes the most sense for them." Health insurers understand that the major value proposition for their services will be bringing a value-driven organizational discipline to the fragmented health system. In working with more organized health systems and physician groups, they can contribute value through their information systems, data, product knowledge, marketing, sales, and brand as well as their financial expertise and resources.

These tailored, narrow networks can be controversial. Ultimately, the value to the consumer must be demonstrated. In some communities, the value of narrow networks will also need to be demonstrated to politicians and regulators. There will be an ongoing dynamic between network design, choice, and cost management.

Vertical integration of insurers with providers is increasing. Full integration with insurer ownership of providers is situational. Just as with providers integrating into the insurance business, there are unintended consequences. The opportunities for full integration are market-specific. The key is the market density of the insurer's covered population. Is there enough patient volume to support the provider's overhead? Is there consumer desire for an insurance product that restricts provider choice? Is there enough cost savings to create an advantage? What is the competitive reaction of the other providers in the market?

It is possible that collaboration between large insurers and large provider organizations will form the basis for the narrow networks bearing risk. The success of the collaboration will ultimately be determined by consumer value. The ability to align incentives producing value will require skill, knowledge, and organizational agility. The insurance products will be expected to grow and produce new patient volume for the providers. As utilization declines from more effective medical management, providers must "make it up in volume." Managing this "equation of expectations" (providers expect more volume for lower pricing or more effective utilization, so their overall revenue stays the same or increases) in an era of value-based payments will be a challenge. Competition between networks in markets will motivate all participants. The speed of market change is a key determinant of these vertical integration strategies for insurers.

In addition to network management, many health insurers are aggressively pursuing the $n - 1$. Consumers increasingly look to insurers to be providers of information for effective and informed purchase of health services. Health insurers are creating transparency of pricing and quality information, as well as the tools to use information, allowing consumers to manage their high-deductible health plans successfully. In addition, they create the healthcare marketplace by organizing networks of physicians and creating consumer health products. As they acquire information through these transactions, further refinement of network, pricing, and product can be achieved.

The exchange market places are changing the dynamic for insurers. The standardization, comparability, and transparency of exchanges create a need to refine product offerings. Dr. Kaveh Safavi, global managing director for Accenture's healthcare business, speaks to research that shows that, within five years, 20 percent of Americans will purchase benefits from a public or private exchange, as noted in Figure 6.

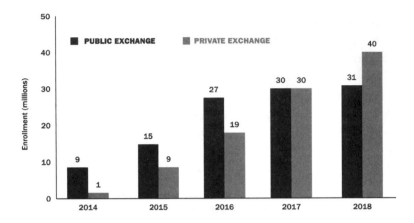

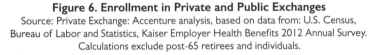

Figure 6. Enrollment in Private and Public Exchanges
Source: Private Exchange: Accenture analysis, based on data from: U.S. Census,
Bureau of Labor and Statistics, Kaiser Employer Health Benefits 2012 Annual Survey.
Calculations exclude post-65 retirees and individuals.

This means insurance companies will be marketing head-to-head with other insurance companies in a standardized market. This is analogous to the Amazon marketplace. The consumer will have easy-to-use, visually understandable, and comprehensive options to purchase their health insurance. Research suggests that consumer choice may mitigate the concern about moving to a high-deductible plan. As these highly transparent public and private marketplaces grow, the ability to clearly demonstrate differential value to the consumer will be an issue for insurers.

The telecommunications industry has similarities. The ability to create market distinction with the core business was diminished with increased transparency and technological advancement. Their move has been to create differential value by moving into the content space, such as entertainment.

Health insurers are also looking beyond the products and the networks to seek and create value for the consumer. Insurers have set up wellness centers and wellness tools for consumers. These range from online tools to fitness centers in malls to coaches who are willing to work out with individuals. Many health insurers are developing personal relationships with consumers to improve their health. Health insurers have been quick to understand the n = 1 and the importance of connecting to unique individuals, particularly as the market moves to more and more individual products.

The insurer's brand is important for individuals. It is the trusted source of information, the network of providers, the benefit structure, the wellness programs, as well as the financial system to seamlessly pay for the services. Providers might be viewed in a transactional way. As has occurred in other industries, as the n = 1 consumer purchases, organizations with the closest relationship to the individual have the brand advantage. This could result in disintermediation of the traditional relationships between the consumer and a service provider.

This blurring of boundaries between insurers and providers for closeness of brand to unique individuals will be a source of competition in the future. These issues will play out on a local level based on a multitude of factors. The questions asked by insurers and providers should be informed by the history of how branding and closeness to the consumer have played out in other industries.

Many health insurers are moving into other innovative businesses, which can have an impact on healthcare costs and quality. Health insurers' strong financial position and clarity of strategic intent provide them with significant advantages in attracting and accelerating innovative ideas. Significant opportunities are being developed in predictive analytics, apps, mobile technology, and clinical research. At least one leader of venture capital has said that they would prefer to invest in health insurance innovation or consumer innovation, as opposed to provider systems, because of easier adoption by consumers and insurers.

Health insurers are well positioned for transformation. They have the financial strength, data, customer focus and infrastructure to add value to the n = 1. Their increasingly significant role in government programs and with the individual market will be key to their success. Their effective relationships with the government at the federal level will continue to serve them well as healthcare is increasingly politicized. They will develop significant partnership arrangements with providers to add value in the delivery system. In five years, visionary and well-capitalized health insurance companies will look nothing like they do today.

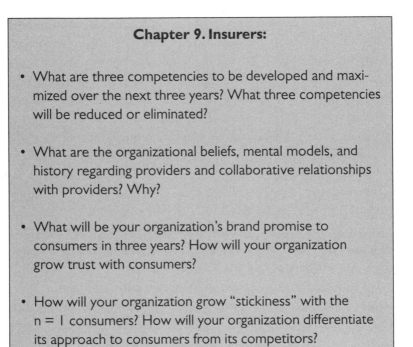

Chapter 9. Insurers:

- What are three competencies to be developed and maximized over the next three years? What three competencies will be reduced or eliminated?

- What are the organizational beliefs, mental models, and history regarding providers and collaborative relationships with providers? Why?

- What will be your organization's brand promise to consumers in three years? How will your organization grow trust with consumers?

- How will your organization grow "stickiness" with the n = 1 consumers? How will your organization differentiate its approach to consumers from its competitors?

CHAPTER 10

New Entrants

New organizations based on digitization and disruptive innovations are being spawned. Transference of risk and new reimbursement incentives create new business model opportunities. Existing organizations will continue to expand their mix of services, as well as to vertically and horizontally integrate. New entrant startups are carving niches in healthcare. As with every other industry sector, new market entrants see opportunity. They feel passionate about the need to disrupt existing ways and enable change.

Many of the entrepreneurs in the healthcare sector have an almost religious zeal for change, based on their belief that healthcare must be improved. A surprising number have personal stories about the inadequacies of the healthcare "system" as their motivation for disruption. Figure 7 shows the tremendous increase in venture funding for digital health companies.

At times of powerful transformational forces, as is the case in healthcare today, there will be many new entrants. In fact, as noted in Figure 8, nearly one-half of Fortune 50 companies are new entrants in healthcare. As reimbursement incentives change from the fee-for-service structure of the past, the opportunities for new entrants will expand dramatically. They will have different business models and new competencies. Their business models are unencumbered by the politics and requirements of the old delivery models.

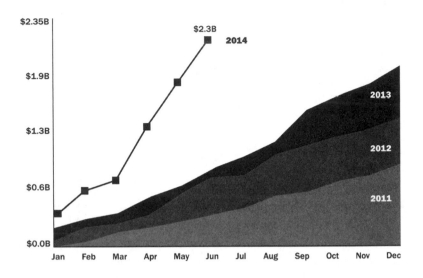

Figure 7. Venture Funding for Digital Health Companies, 2011–2014 to date
Source: Rock Health funding database. Note: Only includes deals > $2M.

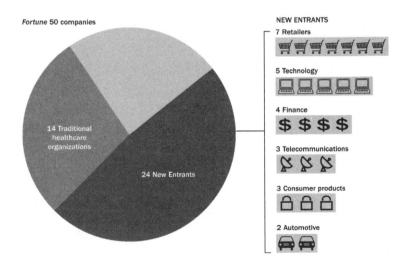

Figure 8. *Fortune* 50 Companies Entering Healthcare
Source: The Health Management Academy Research, *Fortune* 50, 2013.

Recent studies by PwC[41] demonstrate the opportunities for new entrants in the overall revenue for specific services and the potential receptivity of consumers for new means of providing these services. They asked, "How likely would you be to choose these options, if they cost less than the traditional choice?"

Here are the percentages[42] of respondents answering "very likely" or "somewhat likely" (the dollar figures are the annual total U.S. revenue in dollars for that specific service):

- 58.6 percent would use an at-home strep test purchased at a store—$150 million.
- 49.1 percent would have a wound or pressure sore treated at a clinic in a retail store or pharmacy—$796 million (for debridement).
- 54.8 percent would send a general photo of a rash or skin problem to a dermatologist for an opinion—$358 million (for evaluation of contact dermatitis and other minor rashes.)
- 43.6 percent would have an electrocardiogram at home using a device attached to their phone, with results wirelessly sent to their physician—$2.9 billion (for routine EKG).
- 42.6 percent would have a pacemaker or defibrillator checked at home wirelessly by their physician —$110 million (for pacemaker evaluation).
- 41.7 percent would have a urinalysis test at home with the device attached to their phone—$694 million (for urinalysis by dipstick or tablet reagent).
- 36.7 percent would have chemotherapy at home—$3.3 billion (for chemotherapy administration).
- 54.5 percent would check vital signs at home with a device attached to their phone.
- 46.9 percent would check for an ear infection at home using a device attached to their phone.

Over the last two decades, new entrants into healthcare have had variable success. In the mid-'90s, there was a certainty that capitation would be the payment model for managed care. Many organizations sprang up around the business model of "rolling up" medical groups or managing populations or disease states for a fixed amount of money. Organizations such as PhyCor and MedCath were created. In much of the country, healthcare and payment reform didn't evolve as planned. Some new entrant organizations evolved and became successful, while others did not survive. Politicians, the press, and the public vilified managed care. The economy improved, and the healthcare cost crisis was mitigated by transient lower healthcare cost trends in the mid-'90s. The transformational trends did not favor the growth of these innovative companies.

However, many of these companies and their innovative approaches to physician groups survived the challenges and continue in some form today. New entrants invigorate healthcare and create energy for transformation. In the '90s, much of the innovative healthcare thinking was driven by health system concern for new competitors.

The health environment in the near future may be fertile ground for new entrants. This transformation, unlike in the '90s, is driven not only by the change in incentives, but also by the consumer, digitization, and disruptive innovation. The n = 1 will create opportunities for new entrants. In these changing times, the new competitors will come out of the woodwork.

There are two general categories of new entrants: innovative expansion of existing organizations and innovation-enabled organizations. We have selected examples of each to profile.

Innovative Expansion of Existing Organizations

DaVita HealthCare Partners, a medical group, is expanding into a population health management company with potential for global scale. Walgreens, formerly a "drug store company," is evolving into a health company with global scale. These are examples of organizations innovating on an existing platform.

DaVita HealthCare Partners Inc.

On November 1, 2012, DaVita acquired HealthCare Partners for $4.4 billion and renamed itself DaVita Healthcare Partners Inc. (DaVitaHCP). It was a significant strategic step for DaVita, and it was a resounding statement of the value of a physician network that had, by June 2014, nearly 830,000 managed care patients. Let's review the history and strategy of HealthCare Partners.

Medical groups in California have been taking and managing the risk of population healthcare for many decades. These medical groups have become highly proficient at population healthcare, where they take a capitated prepayment. As transformational forces evolved over the last several years, HCP continued to grow. Dr. Robert Margolis, who led the medical group since its founding in 1992, believed HCP had a better way to practice healthcare for patients, payers, and providers.

It is helpful to see the patient's perspective on population healthcare, as delivered by DaVitaHCP, which has decades of experience in delivering population healthcare. It developed sophisticated approaches to care delivery, driven by the data and by the belief in caring for each unique individual. These are examples of case studies from different points on the continuum of care:

Mary is eighty-two years old and has lived in the same Torrance, California, ranch house for the past fifty-five years. Mary had a stroke several years ago, and as a consequence is confined to bed. In the first years after her stroke, she was hospitalized seven times with pneumonia and urinary tract infections from the catheter in her bladder, as well as from congestive heart failure and diabetes. Each hospitalization was distressing, dangerous, and expensive—$3,000 to $4,000 per day.

Several years ago, Dr. Jim began visiting Mary. Her only son was mentally and physically exhausted from the series of emergency hospital visits and knowing that her prior primary care doctor could not provide Mary the type of care she needed.

Dr. Jim is an HCP doctor, board-certified in family medicine. He sees approximately six to eight patients in their homes each day.

One of his patients is Mary.

On a recent visit, Dr. Jim took her blood pressure, checked the healing pressure ulcers that afflict many bed-bound patients, and did a careful inventory of her medications, checking the bottles and tubes she had against the list of medications in the electronic record. It turns out that her mail-order pharmacy service was sending pills she had stopped taking months earlier, so Dr. Jim made a note to tell Mary's case manager.

More than 40 percent of Medicare patients die in the hospital; only 18 to 20 percent of Medicare patients in the HealthCare Partners system die there. At HCP, they are cared for in a more comforting home environment. This is good patient care and is the most compassionate approach to the single biggest driver of healthcare costs, end-of-life care.

On that visit to Mary's house, Dr. Jim noticed a red ulcerated region under Mary's nose where she wears her oxygen prongs at night. Concerned that it might be an early infection, he cultured it with a swab from his bag. He showed Mary how to use one of the antibiotic creams she already had to prevent the sore from getting worse while he waited for a definitive diagnosis from the laboratory.

Mary has not been hospitalized since becoming one of Dr. Jim's patients a year ago.

Dr. Jim's team of two physicians and four nurse practitioners have divided up the greater Los Angeles area into districts, and have become the temporary primary care physicians to 700 patients who cannot make it to a doctor. Four trained medical assistants and three social workers support their activities from the central office, coordinating services like infusion, wound care, and skilled nursing. These temporary primary care physicians stay in communication with the primary care physicians who took care of these patients before they became homebound and who will resume their care when the patients are able to travel.

What all Dr. Jim's home-visit patients have in common is that they are members of a Medicare managed-care plan that has a full-risk contract with DaVitaHCP. What that means is that DaVitaHCP receives a fixed fee each month for each senior citizen enrolled in the plan, equivalent to what Medicare would pay for a similar patient. DaVitaHCP is responsible for paying for all their medical care, from doctors' visits to hospitalizations to surgeries.

This payment system creates a remarkable alignment of interests: It is irrelevant that Dr. Jim's home-visit unit would lose massive amounts of money in a traditional fee-for-service system. Dr. Jim's job isn't to see a lot of patients; his job is to take great care of Mary and patients like her. His team ensures that they remain healthy and stay out of the hospital. This saves DaVitaHCP thousands of dollars each time a hospitalization is prevented. Another additional benefit is that Mary's son's health has also improved because of the support to his mother.

The alignment of incentives and the care design around the n = 1 unique individual assures that the healthcare system benefits from the more effective use of the expensive resources. Another case example is the approach DaVitaHCP takes to discharge planning and hospitalization.

Just as Dr. Jim and other DaVitaHCP clinicians work to keep patients out of the hospital, a highly organized team of hospitalists, doctors who do nothing but care for patients admitted to the hospital, works on getting patients home as quickly as possible.

For anyone who has been hospitalized with a serious condition that isn't life-threatening, the seemingly slow pace of hospital-based diagnosis and treatment can be maddening. Many hospitals turn in impressive results when speed matters, but when there is not a sense of urgency, hospitals can function at a different speed. Hours can pass between when a physician orders a CT scan and when the CT scan is performed. More hours pass before a radiologist interprets the CT scan images, and more hours pass between when the radiologist's report is available and when the physician who ordered the test in the first place has a chance to review the findings and plan treatment. As hours blend into days, the costs and the risks of being in the hospital add up.

DaVitaHCP's response to this is a specialized team of 100

hospitalists deployed at the thirty Los Angeles-area hospitals where HealthCare Partners admits patients. These hospitalists are not above paging a radiologist to interpret an MRI that was recently completed, or going to a bedside to make sure that an ordered medication is promptly hanging on the IV pole. As a result, the average length of stay for DaVitaHCP's patients is 3.3 days, compared to the national average of approximately six days. At $3,000 per day, that's a savings of more than $8,000 each time a DaVitaHCP patient is hospitalized. The averted risk to the patients from prevented iatrogenic injury is additive to this savings.

When patients go home from the hospital, DaVitaHCP has an entire team dedicated to making sure that they don't need to be readmitted. It is well known in medicine that the patient at highest risk for being admitted to the hospital is the patient who was just discharged. Patients forget to take their medications (or don't have someone to pick them up at the pharmacy on their behalf). They forget to make a follow-up appointment with their primary care doctor. They ignore the signs that they are deteriorating and don't get seen by their doctor until they are so sick that another hospitalization is the only option.

DaVitaHCP tackles the readmissions by managing the logistics of the discharge process. At DaVitaHCP, a team of a dozen professionals call patients the day after discharge to check on them. They call primary care doctors to make follow-up appointments. They weave their way through the physician's front office "phone tree." They patiently wait on hold when the primary care physician's receptionist is busy. They confirm that in-home visits from wound-care nurses and IV infusionists have started and medications are on hand. Nationwide, the thirty-day readmission rate is approximately 20 percent for non-elective hospital admissions; HealthCare Partners has a 14 percent readmission rate.

In some respects, reducing hospitalizations and shortening the length of time patients' stay in the hospital is the low-hanging fruit of cost-savings in healthcare. Achieving it is one of those accomplishments that seems trivial, but isn't. Healthcare is complex, and outcomes depend on the coordination of dozens of individuals—from the patient to doctors to infusionists to physical therapists.

DaVitaHCP accomplishes this coordination with real-time analysis of data from across its large clinical and financial network; it then deploys organizational systems built on years of experience. It has made a significant investment in preventive care so that patients who might otherwise require hospitalization never get that sick in the first place. That is transformative change.

The transformative n = 1 approach of DaVitaHCP is seen in another case of coordinated care. Mr. Torres and his wife, both seniors, have been members of DaVitaHCP for many years. During that time, both of them enjoyed a healthy lifestyle thanks to regular PCP medical visits, prevention services, and other timely medical interventions. These are particularly important because of Mr. Torres's chronic conditions—diabetes, heart disease, and hypertension.

Gradually, last year, Mr. Torres's health began to worsen. It seemed that with each birthday his chronic diseases became more difficult and complex. His DaVitaHCP PCP turned to a team of special-care experts to help the Torres family. As part of DaVitaHCP's individualized care plan for each patient, patients with high-risk chronic conditions are identified and a specific care management team is introduced rapidly. Their mode of operation is hyper-vigilance.

The care management team delivered Mr. Torres's healthcare very differently. "Instead of seeing many specialists and going from office to office, my doctor and his team revolved around me," Mr. Torres said. "They even provided transportation to the care center because driving was difficult for me. I was at the center of the team, and each doctor or nurse or therapist worked hand in hand to make sure I was getting the care I needed. It's easy to become overwhelmed when your health suffers. We turned to our DaVitaHCP doctor, who coordinated an entire team to help us."

DaVitaHCP's centralized care centers allow for one-stop care for patients with chronic conditions like diabetes, COPD, heart disease, and hypertension. The patient is not a collection of symptoms, but a unique individual, so his care is highly coordinated to allow for warm hand-offs and easy communication between team members. For nine years in a row, DaVitaHCP has been recognized by IHA (Integrated Healthcare Association) for top patient satisfaction, clinical quality, and coordination of complex problems, as well as providing physicians with easy-to-use information technology to accomplish these goals.

"My diabetes went out of control so fast, and now here I had a team that got me back to my old self in just a few days," Mr. Torres said. "My medications were immediately changed, and a diabetic educator was helping not only me but my wife about my diet. Another doctor whom I never met knew all about my health and life when he walked in the room. Soon my blood pressure and heart issues were normal."

Thanks to DaVitaHCP's innovative technology, which allows sharing of patient information between care team members, specialists are aware of real-time medical issues, family history, and even personal information about patients. This creates seamless care coordination and better outcomes.

Mr. Torres said the most important aspect of his care was the fact that he and his wife's stress levels were immediately reduced. "When you get old like me, change and serious illness can turn your peaceful retirement into chaos. Not so with DaVitaHCP. They took the stress off of us. They owned it. I don't know where we'd be without them."

DaVitaHCP's patient-centered care does more than address clinical and medical issues. Warm hand-offs and customer service from each and every touch point along the HCP continuum means better outcomes and satisfied patients.

These case studies demonstrate a transformation of healthcare delivery in a population health model. DaVitaHCP manages the populations with a network that includes non-HCP-employed physicians in the IPA. The elements of care management are intuitive to those involved in healthcare. That is only part of the transformational impact. DaVitaHCP is disruptive because they have built the information and management systems to manage populations at scale.

DaVitaHCP starts from the individual patient, then develops cost-effective and high-quality clinical and care processes that best serve that patient. The clarity of their business model allows them to redefine how care is given. Their care delivery processes will reach out to a patient and treat them in more economical and convenient care settings. They have a powerful belief in team medicine. They partner and purchase hospital services and do not believe they need to own expensive and capital-intensive facilities in order to deliver their care.

The DaVitaHCP team believes the keys to delivering population-based healthcare are:

- A strong and well-aligned physician and care team culture
- Deep usable clinical and administrative data regarding the population
- A superior data warehouse and predictive modeling capability
- A culture of full transparency with continuous improvement in quality, outcomes, and patient satisfaction
- Strong teams of administrative leadership and physician leadership at all levels of the organization
- Aligned incentives at all levels

Regarding the acquisition by DaVita, the strength of the publicly traded company allows for the capitalization of further care process improvements, digitization, and expansion. DaVitaHCP has expanded from three to five states over the last few years. They believe theirs is a global market. The transformative forces of healthcare are shifting incentives toward population-based healthcare. Innovative organizations like DaVitaHCP have experience, vision, scale, and organizational structure to take advantage of the market changes.

A key part of the DaVitaHCP business model is its ability to engage physicians who are not employed by DaVitaHCP. These physicians are part of the DaVitaHCP contracting network. The ability to have these physicians in an expanded network, according to Dr. Margolis, provides DaVitaHCP with the ability to:

- Provide much greater patient choice, for instance, big clinic sites versus local doctor offices;

- Possess growth potential without big fixed-cost structure (such as Kaiser might have);
- Work with physicians as trusted partners and customers of DaVitaHCP's capabilities.

DaVitaHCP, even with its proven track record of managing population healthcare, must continue to innovate and evolve. Their care management processes are not proprietary and in most instances make sense from a good medical care standpoint. There is no question that other medical groups and health systems perform similar care management. So what is it that makes DaVitaHCP a disruptive new market entrant? If the future is population healthcare, what are the elements of DaVitaHCP that will be successful? They focus on the areas of highest cost in healthcare: hospital, end-of-life, chronic illness, specialty physician services, and poor hand-offs and communication. How will health systems achieve similar effectiveness?

Walgreens

Walgreens's stated purpose is: "to help people get, stay, and live well." Walgreens's vision is to be the first choice in healthy and daily living for everyone in America—and beyond.

The CEO of Walgreens, Greg Wasson, notes that 70 percent of Americans who visit the emergency room do not have or utilize a primary care physician. In addition, he notes, there are emerging health-care delivery models resulting from the shift from fee-for-service to pay for performance.

Their statistics are impressive: 8,200 health and daily-living destinations (retail stores and clinics), 70,000 professionals, 400 health-care clinics, 370 worksite clinics, and two central specialty care centers. They lead with their core competence of pharmacy services. They've enhanced the consultative services of their pharmacists, so that now the pharmacist can be a trusted "go-to" advisor for the customer. They continue to expand their industry-leading presence in the immunization market.

Walgreens's healthcare clinics in their pharmacies provide services such as wellness and prevention, treatment of minor illnesses, and monitoring and management of chronic illness. In addition, they have healthcare's largest on-site work clinic presence. They are continuously innovating their delivery offerings and have recently completed a partnership with another innovator, the laboratory service disruptor Theranos, which will be discussed later. In addition to care delivery in the pharmacies and at work sites, they have the nation's largest home infusion network. They are intent on developing strategic partnerships with providers and insurers throughout the country.

Walgreens, anticipating the transformational forces, is expanding its services in healthcare delivery and patient care management. Their closeness to the customer and their strong brand facilitate the continued expansion of their services. Their scale combined with digitization and a long presence in predictive analytics within the pharmacy business creates potential for ongoing disruptive innovation. The change in the assumption of risk resulting in the retail purchase of healthcare continues to drive opportunity for Walgreens.

How will the entrance of Walgreens into care delivery impact your health system?

What is the importance of brand to the individual seeking healthcare?

If you were Walgreens, how would you continue to evolve the delivery model?

How does this compare to and contrast with insurance companies moving into a branded relationship to individuals? The retail pharmacies and insurance companies have large data management resources; how does this create opportunities and threats for health systems and physician groups?

Innovation-Enabled Organizations

Theranos is a highly disruptive laboratory services company. Castlight Health is devoted to providing healthcare consumers with education and pricing transparency.

Theranos

Theranos is an innovative laboratory services company enabled by disruptive technology. Former Secretary of State George Schultz, a board member, has described its young CEO, Elizabeth Holmes, as the next Steve Jobs. The board of Theranos may be the most accomplished board in U.S. corporate history, according to *Fortune*'s Roger Parloff. It includes Henry Kissinger, Sam Nunn, and Bill Frist in addition to Schultz.

Theranos has eighty-two (sixteen approved) U.S. patents and 189 (sixty-six approved) foreign patent applications. Over the last decade, the company has perfected technology that allows the painless collection of a few drops of blood from the patient. These minute samples are quickly analyzed and are rapidly conveyed to the cloud, then to the provider and subsequently to the patient.

The cost of the diagnostic lab services is set at 50 percent of the Medicare fee schedule, which significantly undercuts most laboratories' pricing today. According to their website, Theranos charges $5.35 for a CBC with differential and $4.82 for electrolytes. They publish all their pricing and quality information publicly.

The proprietary blood-drawing techniques do not require venipuncture. This blood sampling can occur in many different settings. It has strong satisfaction for individuals who have required frequent blood draws or those with difficulty providing samples. This significant price advantage and speed of service demonstrates how n = 1 requirements will be met: more cheaply, more easily, and faster.

The disruptive technological innovation and digitization, focused

"This CEO is Out for Blood"
by Roger Parloff (@rparlof) June 12, 2014, 7:37 a.m. EDT

Theranos runs what's called a high-complexity laboratory, certified by the federal Centers for Medicare & Medicaid Services (CMS), and it is licensed to operate in nearly every state. It currently offers more than 200–and is ramping up to offer more than 1,000–of the most commonly ordered blood diagnostic tests, all without the need for a syringe.

Theranos's tests can be performed on just a few drops of blood, or about 1/100th to 1/1,000th of the amount that would ordinarily be required–an extraordinary potential boon to frequently tested hospital patients or cancer victims, the elderly, infants, children, the obese, those on anticoagulants, or simply anyone with an aversion to blood draws. Theranos phlebotomists–technicians licensed to take blood–draw it with a finger stick using a patented method that minimizes even the minor discomfort involved with that procedure. (To me, it felt more like a tap than a puncture.)

The company has performed as many as 70 different tests from a single draw of 25 to 50 microliters collected in a tiny vial the size of an electric fuse, which Holmes has dubbed a "nanotainer." Such a volley of tests with conventional techniques would require numerous tubes of blood, each containing 3,000- to 5,000-microliter samples.

The fact that Theranos's technology uses such microscopic amounts of blood should eventually allow physicians far greater latitude when ordering so-called reflex tests than they have previously enjoyed. With reflex testing, the physician specifies that if a certain test comes up abnormal, the lab should immediately perform follow-up tests on the same sample to pinpoint the cause of the abnormality. Reflex testing saves patients the time, inconvenience, cost, and pain of return doctor visits and additional blood draws.

continued

continued

The results of Theranos's tests are available within hours–often matching the speed of emergency "stat" labs today, though stat labs, which are highly inefficient, can usually perform only a limited menu of maybe 40 tests.

Most important, Theranos tests cost less. Its prices are often a half to a quarter of what independent labs charge, and a quarter to a 10th of what hospital labs bill, with still greater savings for expensive procedures. Such pricing represents a potential godsend for the uninsured, the insured with high deductibles, insurers, and taxpayers. The company's prices are set to never exceed half the Medicare reimbursement rate for each procedure, a fact that, with widespread adoption, could save the nation billions. The company also posts its prices online, a seemingly obvious service to consumers, but one that is revolutionary in the notoriously opaque, arbitrary, and disingenuous world of contemporary healthcare pricing.

Precisely how Theranos accomplishes all these amazing feats is a trade secret. Holmes will only say–and this is more than she has ever said before–that her company uses "the same fundamental chemical methods" as existing labs do. Its advances relate to "optimizing the chemistry" and "leveraging software" to permit those conventional methods to work with tiny sample volumes.

"Consumerizing this healthcare experience is a huge element of our mission," Holmes says at our first meeting in April, "which is access to actionable information at the time it matters." In our conversations over the next two months, she comes back to that phrase frequently. It is the theme that unifies what had seemed to me, at first, a succession of diverse, disparate aspects of her vision.

Today people might have their blood tested once a year, she explains. They get a snapshot of certain key values and learn whether they are "in range"–that is, statistically normal–or "out of range." But if they were tested more often, they would begin to see a "movie" of what's going on inside them. Sudden, rapid changes in some protein concentration–even when technically still in range–could tip off the doctor that something was amiss, and do so before it was too late to address the problem. (Theranos plans soon to display results in a way that maps them against all previous results from tests it has performed for that patient.)

"The movie goal is absolutely core to what we're working to do," she says. "When you have that trend, it is a much more meaningful clinical data set for the physician to use."

She knows that, she says, "because we've seen it." She's referring to the fact that since 2005 Theranos has been doing work for major pharmaceutical companies, including Pfizer and GlaxoSmithKline, that are conducting clinical drug trials. Early on it was a way for the company, working under confidentiality agreements, to stealthily refine its technology while earning revenue needed to build out infrastructure. Theranos would test drug-trial subjects three times a week–which wouldn't have been feasible using venipuncture–and catch adverse drug effects quickly, before they became dangerous.

"We're building an early-detection system," she explains. "I genuinely don't believe anything else matters more than when you love someone so much and you have to say goodbye too soon. I deeply believe it has to be a basic human right for everybody to have access to the kind of testing infrastructure that can tell you about these conditions in time for you to do something about it. So that's what we're building."

This story is excerpted from the June 30, 2014 issue of *Fortune*.

on the consumer, has the potential to revolutionize laboratory services.

In an article in the *Wall Street Journal* (September 8, 2013), Holmes said, "We're here in Silicon Valley, inside the consumer technology world, and what we think we are building is the first consumer healthcare technology company. Patients are empowered by having better access to their own health information and then by owning their own data."

Theranos has developed a relationship with Walgreens and is seeking relationships with physicians and other providers. Holmes states that her long-term goal is to have Theranos services "within five miles of virtually every American home."

The "lab-on-a-chip" technology is the focus of a multitude of innovators. The technology of microfluidics and nanofluidics is exploding as complementary knowledge from multiple fields is brought together. Theranos is the early entrant into a diagnostic laboratory industry that will soon be full of disruptive entrants. There will be regulatory, business model, and competitive challenges for Theranos. They will continue to evolve. The fact is that "the genie is out of the bottle." The vision of Elizabeth Holmes and Theranos is for a different healthcare experience.

Theranos is one of many disruptive innovators creating new business models and new competitors in healthcare. Theranos has kept their technology a tightly guarded secret. Some observers question their ability to do what they claim to do. It is a moot point. If not them, it will be someone else. There are other organizations working on similar technologies. Theranos is a prime example of vision enabled by digitization and disruptive scientific innovation to serve n = 1.

How will your organization evaluate Theranos or others with similar technology?

What is the impact on your business model? What are the opportunities?

What is your competitive analysis of the consumer's response to the technology? Should you be an early adapter, or late? Is there a competitive challenge if Walgreens widely commercializes the consumer channel first?

Castlight Health

Castlight is a disruptive new entrant based on consumer health-care education and transparency.

Castlight's Solution in its IPO S–1

Our Solution

We have developed a new category of cloud-based software that enables enterprises to gain control over their rapidly escalating healthcare costs. Our Enterprise Health-care Cloud offering transforms a massive quantity of complex data, which we obtain from a diverse array of internal and external sources, into transparent and useful information for employers, and their employees and families.

We deliver this powerful offering through a suite of innovative applications that enables employers to engage their employees with personalized, actionable information, implement highly tailored benefit designs and integrate their other systems, applications and programs. These applications are delivered to our customers, and their employees and families, via our cloud-based offering and leverage consumer-oriented design principles that drive engagement and ease of use. In addition, as more customers use our applications and our database grows, the depth and breadth of our offering improves, increasing the value we can deliver to employers, and their employees and families.

The key dimensions of our Enterprise Healthcare Cloud offering include:

Extensive Data Foundation

Our Enterprise Healthcare Cloud offering integrates, organizes and normalizes data from across the fragmented

continued

---

continued

and complex healthcare landscape. Much of this information has been traditionally difficult to obtain and, in many cases, inaccessible to employers, their employees and families, and benefit providers. Our offering has successfully scaled to aggregate more than a billion healthcare claim transactions from public and private data sources, which include our customers' health plans and other third parties, and combines these data with healthcare benefit information, clinical practice guidelines, user-generated data and the consumer behavior data of our users. We then structure these data, allowing us to map personalized cost information by region and individual service providers for a broad range of healthcare and physician services and medical products. We combine these pricing data with clinical quality and patient experience information from national, regional and user-generated sources to deliver service-specific quality metrics across a broad range of providers in the United States. Our consumer healthcare database allows our suite of applications to deliver transparency on cost and quality of healthcare services to an otherwise opaque market.

Sophisticated Analytics

Over the last four years, our team of leading engineers, economists and clinicians has developed proprietary data science techniques and robust capabilities to process and analyze our extensive data foundation and compute cost and quality data for thousands of healthcare services and products. Our offering transforms unstructured data from disparate sources into actionable information on price and quality of healthcare services. In addition, we employ predictive modeling to identify patients at risk for needing particular services and estimate their future cost of care. We also use epidemiologic analytics to personalize

continued

continued

recommendations for employers for specific benefits programs in which they should invest based on the health characteristics of their populations. Our offering uses this analytics engine to calculate costs and identify patterns of inefficient behavior for large populations of employees and their families, thereby enabling employers to take actions to optimize benefit plans, reduce inefficient outcomes and foster behavioral change.

Personalized Cost, Quality and Benefit Information

We simplify the healthcare decision-making process for employees and their families by providing highly relevant, personalized information that encourages informed choices before, during and after receiving healthcare. We utilize a real-time interface to securely aggregate the employee's latest medical spending information. By combining these data with medical claims history, benefit plan information, the available provider network and robust search capabilities, we can deliver a highly personalized healthcare shopping experience that illuminates both the employee's specific out-of-pocket costs and the portion of the medical expense paid by their employer. In addition, we deliver personalized benefit and clinical information, as well as specific alerts about lower cost medical and pharmaceutical options, avoidance of unnecessary services and preventative care recommendations. By empowering employees and their families with the ability to simultaneously search price, quality and relevant content on healthcare services and providers, we enable them to make informed "market-based" decisions that avoid excessive prices and low quality or unnecessary care, creating significant value for employers.

Castlight describes itself as "a care management platform designed to transform the healthcare experience for employer and their employees. Castlight helps employees reduce spending and improve the quality of care at the same time. They present personalized cost alongside quality information to help employees get high-value care." The tools, which demonstrate provider pricing and quality, are available on the web, through mobile technologies, and via phone.

If the patient seeks information on emergency-room visits for certain diagnoses, a prompt will inform her regarding urgent-care clinics. The same types of alerts inform patients about generic drugs over brand-name drugs. In addition to the transparency of pricing and quality, they offer integrated clinical education. This education helps patients understand their care options and plan their healthcare services appropriately. All these tools are portable, which enables patients to be prudent consumers of healthcare resources.

Castlight tools on the web and mobile platforms create the transparent consumer experience necessary for retail healthcare. Castlight uses predictive analytics to continually refine the information that is given to consumers. They are just beginning the measurement and reporting of cost and quality information to consumers.

Where they have achieved penetration, Castlight has had an impact on healthcare providers. It only takes one experience of a physician losing a patient to another physician because of a procedure's overall price to make a lasting impression on that physician. These "lost patient" experiences have generated energetic dialogue between physicians, medical groups, facilities, and hospitals.

Castlight's tools are disruptive and innovative. Digitization, predictive analytics, mobile computing technology, and new payment models enable these tools. There will be many other entrants into this space as retail medicine grows. These tools will rapidly gain higher levels of sophistication. Insurance companies are already competitive in the same area. Entrepreneurs who have developed competencies for empowering individual consumers in other sectors see healthcare as a massive opportunity.

Chapter 10. New Entrants:

- What are the scenarios or guidelines for your organization to compete, partner, or buy a new entrant in the market?

- New entrants will generally cannibalize your organization's existing business. What are three implications for your decision-making based on this? What three areas (such as laboratory services) of your organization are most vulnerable to new entrants? Why? What, if anything, should you do?

- For each of the new entrants in the book, what are three lessons your organization can learn? How do you create a question-and-learning session with senior management? Up-and-coming leaders? The board?

PART V

A Key Constituency

The board of every healthcare organization will be challenged by the changes driven by the $n = 1$. Physician groups, insurers, biotechnology, pharmaceutical companies, and health systems will all be increasingly changed by the transformative forces. Boards must work closely with management to understand the choices management must make in a new environment. The most effective boards will partner with management to find opportunity in the transformation and serve the $n = 1$ in new, value-driven ways.

CHAPTER 11

The Board's Role

As health systems continue to consolidate and grow, their boards of trustees are evolving. New models of governance are developing that are more suited to large, complex organizations. At the same time, boards must monitor the environment and develop strategies with management to ensure that their health system adapts. The boards of all healthcare companies are faced with the same challenges.

Boards interface with the community, providing advice, wisdom, and judgment to assist the CEO and the health system. This is particularly important during times of major transformation. Different boards have different constituencies. For example, not-for-profit health system boards provide the perspective of the community; physician boards represent the professional constituency of the medical group; and investor-owned boards represent shareholders within the context of operating a healthcare company with community responsibilities.

Not-for-profit health system boards have a unique position because many board members are volunteers or receive very little compensation for serving. They are governing large and complex organizations, representing the community and its many constituencies. They may vary dramatically in understanding of healthcare—how it is organized, financed, and delivered. Boards must act in the best interests of the health system and the community. The speed and complexity of transformation challenges boards of all healthcare companies.

Like other aspects of healthcare, "If you've seen one health system board, you've seen one health system board." The history of the health system, its ownership, and the demands and needs of communities all play into the diversity of health system management and governance models.

The governance models of medical groups are also diverse, based on their heritage, composition, and size. Frequently, there is a close link between board membership and representation of the professional group. In these professional representational models, there is a high level of accountability of the board to the professionals. Communication by the board to the physicians is a high priority. This can be challenging because of the workload and distraction of practicing physicians. The physicians may not be able to grasp issues that may have profound impact on them. This is not because they are incapable, but because they feel consumed with caring for their patients.

Evolution of Governance Model

The evolution of governance responsibilities in not-for-profit health systems, from being a trustee of a single hospital to that of a large, multi-billion dollar health system, is particularly dramatic. A hospital trustee might be a local businessperson or retired executive fulfilling her desire for community service by serving on a hospital board. Priorities include fundraising for new programs or buildings, monitoring medical staff issues, and providing support and oversight for the operations of the hospital.

The board members of large health systems, who may have begun as hospital trustees, now have oversight of complex vertically and horizontally integrated health systems. In fact, of the largest 100 not-for-profit health systems, more than one-third would rank in the Fortune 1000 if they were publicly-traded companies.[43] Multistate or multi-site health systems are complex, and require the board member to be responsible for the overall performance of the health system, including system-level services provided to each of the individual facilities and operations within the health system.

Consolidation involving vertical or horizontal integration creates the potential for a change in board composition. This may lead to a change in board dynamics and culture. This change can either nourish or disrupt the functioning of the board. This dynamic needs to be managed carefully so it is a nourishing change. Agreement from all parties on governance models is a good start. Clear management and governance matrices, including subsidiary boards, should document the roles of decision-making throughout the management and governance structure. This clear accountability for decision-making underlies successful consolidation in other industries as well as health systems.

Board Composition

The composition of boards is in the process of evolving to a competency model rather than a community representation model. Those competencies are identified by the governance committee of the board, in partnership with the CEO, and relate to the current and future needs of the organization. Health systems will often develop and manage a pool of potential candidates who possess desired competencies.

Competencies such as insurance, information systems, marketing, retail, government relations, and communications are being sought by boards, along with diversity of age, gender, race, and perspective.

Given the size and complexity of large health systems, the competency model and the time required, a growing number of large not-for-profit health systems are compensating board members.

Not-For-Profit Board Responsibilities

Four broad areas of not-for-profit board responsibility deserve particular attention.

- *Selection of the CEO.* This is the most important priority of the board. The board maintains a productive relationship with the CEO through clarity of expectations. Goals, objectives, incentives, compensation, and evaluation of the CEO are key responsibilities of any board, not-for-profit health systems included. Boards develop a manageable list of CEO performance objectives drawn from the strategy of the health system. These should serve as the focus of the ongoing discussions between the CEO and the board.

- *Strategy.* The board must own strategy. This was much easier for a trustee of a single hospital than one for a large multi-hospital system in today's dynamic environment. Since boards meet only periodically and are not composed entirely of healthcare experts, a major priority of the CEO is to arrange ongoing internal and external education for the board. They must monitor and anticipate the effect of environmental trends. For example, most board members can identify how the unique individual, n = 1, is transforming their own business and their lives. How can this experience in their business be converted to strategy for the health system?

- *Strategic framework and mental models.* Board decision-making in a complex and rapidly transforming industry like healthcare requires a sound conceptual framework. The board member's mental model of the health system is critical. Is it still the hospital? Is it still fee-for-service? Is it still inpatient? The board must develop a different mental model for the health system's role in the community in population healthcare. What is it? Developing a consistent language and description of these models is helpful to board members.

- *Talent development.* The board will work closely with the CEO to ensure talent development by the organization. The board will be informally evaluating senior management on an ongoing basis and discussing their impressions. Strategy discussions will include consideration of required new talent. Ongoing consideration of organizational talent development and compensation strategies will assist the CEO. Board members should bring their professional experience in this area to the board to assist the CEO.

How Do We Make Money?

Not-for-profit boards may not be clear about the financial drivers of the health system. Our research shows that successful CEOs and boards continually discuss finances to the level of granularity of the major contributors to profitability by program line, line of business, payer, and perhaps geographic location. This is a strategic discussion, not just oversight of financial performance.

Discussions of profitability and cash flow provide the foundation for meaningful discussion about the strategic and capital plan. The ultimate goal is to make the budget the actualization of the strategy of the health system. Clearly, the CEO, CFO, and senior management must work hand in hand with the board to ensure nuanced understanding of the health system's finances. The understanding of revenue generation will increase the relevance of the strategic planning process.

Strategy is sometimes defined by what you *don't* do, rather than what you *do*. For example:

- What will our mix of clinical services be in the future? What will we stop doing?
- How do we serve the community differently in the future? What won't we do, that we do now?
- What are the skill sets we need in the future? What are the skill sets that we currently have that we will not need?
- What is the future of not-for-profit healthcare? What does that mean for our organization?
- We have been successful as an insurer with underwriting and

benefit design. How will we stop many of those activities and build new capabilities?

The exercise of "what will we stop doing?" can be revealing for the board. Strategy can be clarified when seen in the light of discontinuing the funding of longstanding activities. This is the core of the creative destruction.

Enterprise Risk

Enterprise risk is increasing for large health systems as they grow horizontally and vertically and evolve new strategies. A foundation of risk management should guide the board during times of uncertainty and transition. An annual assessment of risk, by an outside firm and senior management, is considered a board best practice.

The area of risk management in the health systems is evolving and is very different from a few years ago. These changes are best highlighted with a few examples. What is the role of the board in oversight of confidentiality and security of the information gathered about patients and consumers? What if the information is beyond personal health information? What about genomic information? What about information that is about personal behavior and lifestyle, which impacts health and health risk? What should the board know about the partners and vendors of the health system in the big data program? What is the reliability and history of the vendors and partners? What are the goals and objectives of the vendors and partners, and are they consistent with the health system? What are industry best practices on the ethical use of big data?

These issues were unknown a few years ago. They will continue to evolve. Boards must ask incisive questions that help them understand the risks and protect the organization.

Integration and consolidation create similar issues. A health system recently entering the health plan business will want the board to understand medical loss ratios, risk-based capital, incurred but not reported expenses (IBNR), and the insurance regulatory environment for which they are now responsible. Similarly, the insurer with a new medical group will have different issues than they have experienced in the past, such as malpractice, capital expenses, and physician management issues. Boards must take the initiative to work with management to surface the issues that are new to governance oversight.

Board information architecture is a term used to describe the mechanism to transmit performance information effectively from management to the board. The effective communication to the board of the system's complex performance information is a first step in risk management. There is a dynamic tension between how much information a board wants and how much it needs. This varies from board member to board member and requires ongoing internal and external education to standardize board expectations. This is a major role for the chair and the CEO. In these increasingly complex, rapidly evolving organizations, this management of expectation for information is important to keep board members engaged and "out of the weeds."

A method for communicating key performance information to the board, the board information architecture, must be developed. Effective graphic representation of complex data can assist both management and the board in understanding performance. Highly effective information architecture will increase board efficiency, effectiveness, and satisfaction.

Board Best Practices

A CEO succession plan to cover planned or unplanned events is a board best practice. The timing of the CEO's retirement is not the driver of the discussion. The board should allocate time for this ongoing discussion and tie these discussions to its familiarity with senior health system executives. What are the competencies required of the health system's CEO in the future? Will they include clinical skills, knowledge of health insurance, technology, managing complex joint ventures, or "all of the above?" What type of leader will be effective in the health system in the future: servant leader, charismatic leader, thought leader, or other characteristics?

Many health systems provide summarized interim board reports that provide an overview of the health system's performance on the board's top priorities, as well as newsworthy updates. The board will have a commitment, led by the chair, to achieve leading practices and continuous improvement. Annual board self-evaluation and goal-setting are best practices. Integrating new board members through a process of orientation and "social welcoming" pays dividends.

Board chairs maintain a healthy board dynamic and manage board members. They encourage participation, minimize micromanagement, and work closely with the CEO. The best board chairs provide advice and counsel to the CEO and provide feedback on the CEO's style and performance. They also provide feedback to the CEO regarding the board's executive sessions.

The governance of these evolving health systems is an important role for our communities. The transformation occurring is shaping the future of healthcare. The individuals involved in governance of the emerging, integrated health systems find their work challenging and invigorating. This is a place where the unique individual, n = 1, *as a board member*, has the ability to shape the transformation of healthcare.

Chapter 11. The Board

- Does the board understand how the organization makes money today? Does the board understand the management plan for how the organization will make money in three or five years? Is there an understanding of the "bridge strategy," if required, to span the old business model to the new business model?

- What are three areas of the organization that have evolved in the last year that require a discussion of board oversight (e.g., integration, big data, diversification)?

- Are the board members and CEO "up for it"? How do you know? How do they know?

PART VI

Are You Up For
The Challenge?

CONCLUSION

The world is being swept by the impact of the n = 1. This transformational change challenges the orthodoxies and foundations of societies, industries, and professions. Healthcare is beginning this transformation, and healthcare leaders can learn from the experiences of other professions and industries.

The New York Times Example

The *New York Times*, known as the "Gray Lady," is not impervious to transformational change. Let's look at an article from the *Times*[44] for the extent of a report on the need for innovation in newspapers:

> *The Times' report on innovation, put together by a task force headed by A.G. Sulzberger, son of the newspaper's besieged publisher, has implications that resonate far beyond the Times' Midtown Manhattan redoubt. It's must reading for newspaper executives and staffers across the country, and for everyone who cares about journalism.*
>
> *The ambitious report, posted last week by BuzzFeed, finds that the Times is lagging dangerously when it comes to adapting to the digital future. More broadly, it also shines a bright beacon on the severe challenges facing an entrenched business threatened by massive disruption.*
>
> *The report makes clear how hard it is for people and institutions to change what they have been doing for years, regardless of the perceived need to do things differently and the rhetoric that*

accompanies it. And it underscores how difficult it is for established players to compete with nimble new foes unencumbered by the weight of tradition.

The Times has made some great strides in the realm of digital journalism. Its treatment of Snow Fall, its riveting account of a fatal avalanche in Washington State, was a brilliant example of taking advantage of the attributes of the digital platform.

But in many ways, the report states forcefully, the news outlet is hamstrung by its inability to shed the obsession with print habits and customs. A disproportionate amount of time, energy and thinking, for example, is spent on the front page of the next day's newspaper while news is exploding 24/7. The Times' website is organized around print sections.

There is no way to exaggerate the cataclysmic impact the Internet has had on the newspaper industry, once made up largely of monopoly businesses with stratospheric profit margins,

As is often the case with disruptive challenges, the initial industry instinct was to dismiss the Web, to minimize its ramifications, to write it off as a fad. When it became clear that the digital realm was here to stay, the response too often was to take material from the print product and simply dump it onto the web, completely ignoring the differences between the platforms. There was the deep-seated tendency to hold exclusive stories for print rather than posting them when they were available, for fear of "scooping yourself."

Similarly, the tech world's determination to experiment, its willingness to "fail often, fail quickly," is anathema at more established businesses.

The situation is complicated by the fact that while the media world is evolving quickly, and while advertising revenue has dropped at an alarming rate, newspapers still make the bulk of their money from print.

One of the report's key recommendations is creation of a special digital strategy team that could focus entirely on reinvention for the future without the powerful distraction of daily news demands.

It's a good idea. Newspapers across the country would be wise to heed the report's message and redouble (or retriple) their efforts to forge a powerful, truly digital-first approach. Their survival depends on it.

The newspaper and publishing industries are in the midst of disruptive transformation. The professionals in this industry believed themselves to have a special place in society. After all, the U.S. Constitution protects their work. Their compact with society is based on bringing truth and information to the public through print. Newspaper and publishing professionals did not believe the public would abandon them for new nonprint alternatives.

The print media industry believed the standards of the new entrants would be unacceptable to the customer. But new entrants have prospered, with their unconventional and personalized approaches to news coverage. The disappointed newspaper professionals have been humbled. They know they must transform, and, as they do so, they must build on their brand and the public's trust.

n = 1, the Unique Individual

This book described a clear central thesis: personalized expectations and choices are radically changing healthcare, just as they are changing everything else in our world. This power of unique individuals is unrelenting.

The mathematical expression "n = 1" symbolizes the power of the unique individual. This n = 1 is empowered by digitization and scientific innovation. Individuals increasingly demand that products and services fit their personal needs and desires. Because of democratization of information and social networking, they can identify their personalized choices for virtually everything. The results of the n = 1 power are manifest in every aspect of our lives.

Society, government, industry, retail, and media are being transformed, and healthcare is no exception. Healthcare leaders can learn from other leaders, from innovators, and from new entrants in healthcare.

Three major themes of this book capture the essence of this change:

- Unrelenting transformative forces empower the n = 1 to change the world, including healthcare. Leaders must anticipate the impact of these changes. Changes will play out differently, market by market. The forces are constantly evolving. Leaders must be attentive to new opportunities and threats. Leaders must solicit insights and perspectives from many sources to spot trends and opportunities.

- The economics of healthcare are changing dramatically. Financial risk for healthcare services is increasingly being transferred to providers and patients. The resulting change in incentives creates opportunities. These evolving payment models will spur transformation. However, the changes in payment mechanisms are unlikely to occur in a uniform fashion. Thus, the challenges of misaligned incentives will demand courageous leadership for the foreseeable future.

- The leaders of successfully transformed organizations in other industries have confronted reality and asked incisive questions. They have questioned themselves. They have questioned their organizations. Their incisive questions seek to reveal the opportunities being created by change. They have become proficient as an organization in asking incisive questions.

Healthcare Transformation

"Are you up for it?"

Of course you are. The question reflects the gravity and challenge of the task at hand. The earlier article about the *New York Times* describes the difficulty for professionals to engage in creative destruction of the organization they have built, and which provides their livelihood.

What is the mental model necessary for this transformation? What is the organizational culture required? What are the management systems that support change? What kind of board support is required? What are the new and innovative organizational structures? How will new entrants impact the market? The leader must clearly articulate a promising vision for the future, the "future state that best serves our patients." Then the leader must describe the path to the future. Healthcare organizations that don't serve patients, but serve others in healthcare, must ask the same questions. Their customers are changing.

It doesn't make any difference if it's Nokia or the *New York Times*: the need for incisive questions is the same. What questions can healthcare leaders learn from their experiences?

What is different about healthcare? Healthcare is about a uniquely personal and intimate experience. Leaders understand that, in the health system, every day it is the "biggest day" in many people's lives. It can involve a patient or a family member. Life and death, cure and terminal diagnosis, are the purview of the health system. How does the sacred trust of healing differ from the compact of journalism? Consider the admonition of those in journalism and publishing for healers to be cautious about feeling "too special" and irreplaceable. How important is preservation of the sacred trust in healing relationships? Why? How does that impact what you do? Will you preserve it in your health system?

"Calcified hairball" is the term used by some to describe the difficulty for healthcare providers in adopting innovation. The causes of this difficulty are so complex and deep that "calcified hairball" seems an appropriate term, more colorful than Gordian knot. The phrase fits the experience of healthcare leaders. Difficulties are not just with healthcare providers. Vinod Khosla recently interviewed Sergey Brin about Google's potential entry into healthcare. Mr. Brin replied, "It's just a painful business to be in, and the regulatory burden in the United States is so high, that I think it would dissuade a lot of entrepreneurs." (*Wall Street Journal* online, July 28, 2014, opinion, "Let Patients Decide How Much Risk They'll Take," Kevin J. Tracey).

This book has presented many reasons for the "calcified hairball." Among them is the culture of medicine's axiom: "First do no harm."

This is not a bad thing. This culture protects patients, but slows innovation. This is not the culture of tech innovators, who release products before complete refinement and let the market tell them what to fix. Mr. Brin's regulatory experience with his major investment in 23andMe genetics may have influenced his comment. Regulators stopped the company pending further review because of concerns about the safety of individuals' use of personalized genetic sequencing.

Are You Up For It?

Healthcare's challenges will not deter leaders from transforming their organization to serve the n = 1. The same week Mr. Brin expressed his reservations about healthcare, as noted above, Google announced the Baseline Study. Baseline will quantify the detailed physiology of 175 volunteers (much like Larry Smarr). The vast amounts of data captured from these volunteers will be analyzed using Google's "big data" capabilities, producing new insights into health and illness. Google is undeterred by the challenges of healthcare and is committed their mission of adding value. Google's mission is "to organize the world's information and make it universally accessible and useful." They include healthcare in that mission.

Transformative forces are not abating. The economic drivers are not changing. The demand for choice and personalization arising from access to information continues to fuel the evolution of the unique individual, the n = 1.

The challenges can be daunting. Leaders will be faced with situations and opportunities that many in healthcare will insist can't be done. Leaders will say, "Maybe you're right, we can't do this, but if we could, how would we do it?" They ask the questions that open the door to possibilities.

Those leaders who ask the best questions, create the most innovative organizations, and focus on the n = 1 will prevail. They will make healthcare better for all of us.

You are up for it!

ACKNOWLEDGMENTS

Many leaders of healthcare and other sectors have contributed to the content of this book. The new entrants, existing industry members, health insurers, physicians, and health system leaders have been generous in sharing their views. The openness of leaders outside of healthcare is reflective of the importance they place on healthcare's transformation. The discussions and candid dialogue between leaders with many perspectives gives the depth of understanding necessary to discuss this complex topic.

Those who read and contributed to the early manuscripts were patient and diligent, and their input is greatly appreciated: Chris Dawe, Cathy Eddy, Claudia Haglund, Jan Jones, Sherrie Jones, James Garcia, Kavitha Nallathambi, and Hank Walker.

Many leaders with specific expertise and experience made significant contributions to the n = 1 concepts. Many of these leaders contributed time and effort to refine specific issues. They include: Rob Arnold, Mike Butler, Molly Coye, M.D., Jack Friedman, Rod Hochman, M.D., Gus Hunt, Eugene Kolker, Robert Margolis, M.D., Aaron Martin, Pamela Peele, Ph.D., Mark Rosenberg, M.D., and Kaveh Safavi, M.D., J.D.

Members of The Health Management Academy Forums contributed throughout the years by participating in dialogue that generated ideas, shaped them, and tested them against the reality of leading the largest health systems during a time of great transformation.

Ongoing assistance was provided by Caroline Kirk Allen, Cynthia Burr, Azieb Ermias, and Aliza Kwiatek. Sanjula Jain was particularly involved in the book production process.

A special thanks for support from Linda Bisbee and Barbara Koster.

NOTES

[1] "Fifteen Years After Napster: How the Music Service Changed the Industry." *The Daily Beast.com,* June 6, 2014

[2] "Stephen Elop's Nokia Adventure." *Bloomberg Business Week.* June 2, 2011

[3] Academy Fireside chat, CEO Forum, October 2013

[4] Senge, P.M., *The Fifth Discipline* (New York: Doubleday & Co., 1990)

[5] Smallberg, Gerald. "Bias is the Nose for the Story." In *This will make you smarter: New Scientific Concepts to Improve Your Thinking,* John Brockman, ed. (New York: Harper Perennial Digital book, 2012)

[6] Adler-Milstein, Julia; Catherine M. DesRoches, et al. "More than Half of U.S. Hospitals Have at Least a Basic EHR, but Stage 2 Criteria Remain Challenging for Most." *Health Affairs,* August 13, 2014

[7] Ibid.

[8] U.S. Congress, Office of Technology Assessment. *Assessing the Efficacy and Safety of Medical Technologies.* Washington, DC. U.S. Government Printing Office, 1978

[9] Siegler, M. G. *Technomy,* August 4, 2010. Lake Tahoe Technology Conference. Panel Discussion with Eric Schmidt.

[10] Anderson, Chris. "The End of Theory: The Data Deluge Makes the Scientific Method Obsolete." *Wired,* June 28, 2008

[11] Mayer-Schonberger, Victor, and Kenneth Cukier. *Big Data: A Revolution That Will Transform How We Live, Work, and Think* (Kamon Dolan Books e-book, 2013), p. 14

[12] *Science,* March 14, 2014, pp. 1203–1205

[13] Brynjolfsson, Eric, and Andrew McAfee. *The Second Machine Age* (New York: W.W. Norton and Co., 2014), p. 188

[14] Blaser, Martin, M.D. *Missing Microbes* (New York: Henry Holt & Co., 2014), pp. 10–11

[15] Meeker, Mary. "Internet Trends 2014–Code Conference." May 28, 2014 Kleiner Perkins Caufield Byers kpcb.com/internetTrends

[16] Edney, Anna. "FDA Regulators Eye Medical Apps for Mobile Devices." *Bloomberg Business Week*, Sept. 26, 2013

[17] Digital Health Funding. A year in review. January 2, 2014. www.slideshare.net/RockHealth/digital-health-funding-2013-year-in-review

[18] Farr, Christina. *MedCity News*, Dec. 5, 2013

[19] Zimmer, Carl. "Tending the Body's Microbial Garden." *New York Times*, June 17, 2012

[20] "Me, Myself, Us." *Economist*. Aug. 12, 2013

[21] Vishwanat, Dilip. "Study Divides Breast Cancer into Four Distinct Types." *New York Times*, Sept. 23, 2012

[22] Venters, Craig. *Life at the Speed of Light* (New York: Viking, 2013)

[23] Bowden, Mark. "The Measured Man." *Atlantic*, July/August 2012

[24] Centers for Disease Control. *Chart Book of Trends in Health of Americans*, 2007

[25] Joh, Jae Won. *Rock Health*, June 27, 2013

[26] Wolff, Michael, "The Tech Company of the Year is Uber." *USA Today* online, December 22, 2013.

[27] Ries, Eric. *The Lean Startup*. Crown Business Press. 2011 electronic version

[28] Safavi, Kaveh, M.D. Academy presentation, March 29, 2014

[29] Luntz, Frank. *Words That Work: It's Not What You Say, It's What People Hear* (New York: Hyperion, 2007)

[30] Academy charts describing health systems and hospitals

[31] Goold, Michael, and Andrew Campbell. "Desperately Seeking Synergy." *Harvard Business Review*, Sept.–Oct. 1998

[32] Senge, P.M., *The Fifth Discipline* (New York: Doubleday & Co., 1990)

[33] Vladeck, Bruce. "Paradigm Lost: Provider Concentration and the Failure of Market Theory," *Health Affairs* 33, No. 6 (2014), pp. 1083–1087

[34] Porter, Michael E. *Competitive Strategy* (New York: Free Press, 2006)

[35] Mathews, Anna Wilde and Jon Kamp. "WellPoint Names New Chief Executive." *Wall Street Journal* online, February 13, 2013

[36] *Filling the Void, 2013 Physician Outlook and Practice Trends.* Jackson Healthcare, 2013 www.jacksonhealthcare.com/physiciantrends2013

[37] Daniel McCorry, The Heritage Foundation, August 6, 2014

[38] Cosgrove, Toby, M.D. *The Cleveland Clinic Way: Lessons in Excellence from One of the World's Leading Health Care Organizations.* (New York: McGraw Hill, 2014)

[39] Ibid.

[40] JP Morgan Healthcare conference webcast, January 13–16, 2014

[41] "Healthcare's New Entrants: Who Will Be the Industry's Amazon.com?" *PwC*, Health Research Initiative. April 2014 http://pwchealth.com/cgi-local/hregister.cgi/reg/pwc-hri-new-entrants.pdf

[42] Ibid. The annual revenues noted are from the calculated annual revenues received by U.S. providers for commercial claims and Medicare. Approximate national revenue numbers were calculated by applying a national multiplier to these revenue numbers.

[43] *Health Management Academy Research.* Fortune 500, 2014; Fortune 1000 2014.

[44] Sullivan, Margaret. "A Paper Boat Navigating a Digital Sea." *New York Times* online, June 14, 2014

INDEX